Food and Nutrition Economics

Food and Nutrition Economics

FUNDAMENTALS FOR HEALTH SCIENCES

George C. Davis
and
Elena L. Serrano

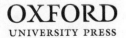

OXFORD
UNIVERSITY PRESS

OXFORD
UNIVERSITY PRESS

Oxford University Press is a department of the University of Oxford. It furthers
the University's objective of excellence in research, scholarship, and education
by publishing worldwide. Oxford is a registered trade mark of Oxford University
Press in the UK and certain other countries.

Published in the United States of America by Oxford University Press
198 Madison Avenue, New York, NY 10016, United States of America.

© Oxford University Press 2016

First Edition published in 2016

Library of Congress Cataloging-in-Publication Data
Davis, George C. (George Carroll), 1960– , author.
Food and nutrition economics : fundamentals for health sciences/George C. Davis
and Elena L. Serrano.
   p. ; cm.
Includes bibliographical references and index.
ISBN 978-0-19-937911-8 (alk. paper)
I. Serrano, Elena L. (Elena Lidia), 1967– , author.   II. Title.
[DNLM: 1. Diet—economics.   2. Nutritional Physiological Phenomena.   3. Choice
Behavior.   4. Food Industry—economics.   5. Food Preferences.   6. Nutritional Status.   QT 235]
RA601
363.19′20681—dc23
2015035605

9 8 7 6 5 4 3

Printed by Webcom, Canada

CONTENTS

PREFACE

Why a Book on Food and Nutrition Economics

Welcome! If you have ever pondered any of the following questions, you are in the right place: Do SNAP benefits (i.e., food stamps) improve diet quality? Are "unhealthy" foods cheaper than "healthy" foods? Will a soft-drink tax reduce caloric intake? Do food labels improve diet quality? What are default effects, and why are they important for nutrition and health? What are the costs and benefits from a nutrition education program? Why don't restaurants sell more nutritious foods? These apparently diverse questions have one thing in common: they are all economic questions. Even a casual reading of popular press or scholarly articles reveals that food, nutrition, and health issues are permeated with economic arguments. Why? Because there is a direct link between economics and food and nutrition.

Simply stated, economics is the study of choices. *Economics* is the study of how individuals make choices subject to constraints, or what health scientists call barriers. *Nutrition* is the study of the nutrients in foods and in the body. So economics informs us on what influences food choices, and nutrition informs us on how those choices affect our health. Both disciplines investigate factors, policies, and interventions that may affect nutrition and health, such as those mentioned in the questions. And yet the communication between economics and health sciences is challenging.

This book is designed to bridge the communication gap between economics and the health science disciplines. While economic considerations are often paramount in analyzing food and nutrition issues, many nutrition and health professionals have very little exposure or training in economic principles. Without an understanding of basic economic principles and mechanisms, it is difficult to analyze or understand the effectiveness of food and nutrition policies or interventions that are designed to operate through economic channels.

The book arose from recognition of this educational gap at Virginia Tech in the nutrition curriculum, especially those in the dietetics track. While students were certainly exposed to economics-based programs, policies, or interventions such as the Supplemental Nutrition Assistance Program (SNAP), soft-drink taxes, or nutrition education programs, they lacked the skills needed to analyze and evaluate the likely impact of these programs. This gap is prevalent in other locations as well. A course was designed at Virginia Tech to meet this need. Of course, we first searched for a book that could be used for the course and found none appropriate. True, the landscape is replete with numerous articles and books that talk about economic topics and nutrition, but most are written by non-economists and none teaches students how *to do* the economics of food and nutrition. This book is designed to be a "travel guide" for the health science student or professional interested in exploring, learning, and conducting a basic economic analysis of food and nutrition problems and not merely reading about findings.

The Intended Audience and Benefits of the Book

Are you intimidated by or find economics challenging? If so, this book is for you. This book is intended for upper-level undergraduates, graduate students, and health professionals with no background in economics but who are serious about learning some economics.

Recognizing that the material may be completely foreign to many, we start from scratch. The book presumes no prior knowledge of nutrition or economics and is designed to be self-contained. All the basic economic principles and tools needed to analyze food and nutrition issues from an economics perspective are explained in the book. Indeed, the material in the book has been well vetted and tweaked as it has been taught for six years to senior dietetic majors at Virginia Tech, most of whom have no economics background.

Economics is first and foremost a way of thinking, a framework for analyzing problems. Upon completion of the book the reader should be able to do the following:

1. analyze the likely impact different economic and environmental factors will have on food consumption, nutrient intake, and certain health outcomes;
2. identify and design economic-based policy instruments that can positively affect food consumption and nutrient intake;
3. identify which policy instruments are likely to be compatible with economic incentives on both the consumer and producer side to improve food and nutrition consumption; and
4. identify the difference between the cost-effectiveness and outcome-effectiveness of different food and nutrition interventions.

After reading and working through the book, the reader should be able to talk intelligently and confidently about the main economic arguments related to food, nutrition, and ultimately health. Furthermore, we believe the book is self-contained enough that a non-economist who has studied and worked through the book could use it to teach a course based on the book.

Additional teaching resources (e.g. test bank, power points) are available at http://www.aaec.vt.edu/people/faculty/davis-george.html

The Structure and Unique Style of the Book

We start Part I on recognizable ground with two overview chapters on nutrition. Part II covers consumer choice economics. We ease into the economics in

Chapter 3 by presenting the major building blocks of neoclassical consumer economics in a very simple setting. Chapters 4 through 8 then focus on adding one new component in each chapter to this foundational framework (e.g., income, then price, then convenience, then information). Chapter 9 gives an overview of behavioral economics, and Chapter 10 demonstrates how the exciting new field of neuroeconomics may help place neoclassical and behavioral economics under one umbrella. Part III covers producer economics. Chapter 11 gives an overview of the food system in the United States, and Chapters 12 and 13 discuss the economics of farm production and then food "beyond the farm gate" production. Part IV covers market-level analysis, where producers and consumers meet. Chapter 14 gives the analytics of supply and demand, and Chapter 15 extends this to the case of horizontally and vertically related markets. Chapter 16 closes the book with an explanation and discussion of cost-identification analysis, cost-effectiveness analysis, and cost–benefit analysis of a nutrient intervention. An Economic Methodology 101 appendix is provided to explain how the economic approach is similar and different from many other sciences.

The general structure for most chapters is to emphasize the importance of the topic, present the economic approach to thinking about the topic, intersperse the text with some examples and think break questions applying the concepts, and conclude the chapter with what has been found in the empirical literature related to the topic.

In terms of style, we use two unique pedagogical devices to enhance learning. First, because the book is designed to help improve communications between health scientists and economists, we have written an ongoing hypothetical conversation between a nutritionist (JP) and an economist (Margaret) that runs throughout the entire book. Each chapter begins with a dialogue between the two about the material to be presented in the chapter. A closing dialogue at the end of the chapter summarizes the material and foreshadows the topic covered in the next chapter.

The second unique style element is how the material in the economic chapters is presented: all material is presented verbally, graphically, and mathematically. Why? A travel metaphor is very useful for explaining this approach. Our experience has been that the main difficulty encountered for those from other disciplines is more the language than the concepts. Many of the concepts are rather intuitive, but the language is foreign. Therefore, think of this as a travel book; a book for adventurers who want to explore and broaden their horizon and learn about the fascinating world that exists at the intersection of nutrition, health, and economics. As in any travel to a foreign land, it helps to be familiar with the native languages. Furthermore, if multiple languages are spoken, some ideas are often easier to express in one language than another.

Economists, and scientists in general, tend to use three languages to communicate: (1) text or spoken language (e.g., English, French), (2) graphical language (e.g., plots, charts), and (3) mathematical language (e.g., algebra, statistics). Each language has advantages and disadvantages; none is a panacea. As different students have different learning styles, different students will probably be more fluent in one of these languages than the other. Consequently, we present ideas in all three languages to facilitate learning (i.e., verbally, graphically, and mathematically). Perhaps you have observed that economists tend to communicate a lot in mathematical languages, and you do not feel very fluent in math. Don't worry. Like all good travel books, this book will provide the translation resources you need to travel effortlessly within the destinations that will be visited. Rest assured, the highest level of mathematics needed or used in this book is middle-school math. In teaching the material to senior-level dietetics majors, we have found that the concepts are not difficult and are often very intuitive, but students just need to "knock off the math rust" and quickly become fluent in the math used in this book. Alternatively, perhaps you have flipped through the book and are put off by the number of graphs. Don't be. Our experience in teaching this material to non-economic students is not that there are too many graphs in economics, but rather that there are not enough! Why? The problem with most graphs in economics textbooks is they seem to presume a lot of background knowledge and often seemed to be pulled out of thin air. We remove the veil and show exactly where all the graphs come from. We proceed sequentially by showing relationships first numerically, then graphically with numbers, then graphically with symbols and some numbers (transition graph), and then finally graphically only with symbols. This pattern will be especially prevalent in the early parts of the book but will diminish as the reader becomes reacquainted with graphs. Once you are fluent in the graphical language, you possess a very powerful tool. Graphs are like conceptual calculators. In the context of our journey, think of the graphs as maps that convey a lot of information in terms of where we have been and where we are going. Remember, a picture is often worth a thousand words!

Before we depart, recognize that as with most worthwhile journeys, there will be periods of intrigue, fascination, questioning, revelation, frustration, bewilderment, and, yes, sometimes even boredom. But at the end of the journey, you will have learned more about the world and yourself. Let the exploration begin!

SUPPLEMENTARY MATERIALS

A major goal in writing this book was to make it as self-contained as possible. However, some may desire more resources and we provide three types at the webpage listed below. First, if you want more help in knocking off the math rust, we provide a mathematical appendix that explains the math and graphs used in the book in more depth. Second, for anyone interested in more application questions, but especially for teachers and students, we provide a test bank of additional questions. We have multiple choice questions, short answer questions, and essay type questions. Finally, we also provide a bank of power points that can be used in either teaching the material or simply studying the material. The questions and the power points have been developed in teaching the course over the past six years.

The weblink for these resources is **http://www.aaec.vt.edu/people/faculty/davis-george.html**

If you go to this link, you will see a link that says "FNE Book". Click on this link and the rest should be self-explanatory. If you have any questions about any of this information feel free to contact us. We would enjoy hearing from you and thanks for your interest.

ACKNOWLEDGMENTS

No book is every really written by just the authors named on the book. We all stand on the shoulders of giants and this book is no different. We would like to thank all at Oxford University Press for their incredible work on this project, but especially Chad Zimmerman for his patience and wonderful editorial guidance through the entire process. Thanks, Chad.

There are too many professional colleagues to thank individually for constructive discussions on the topics covered in this book over the years, but the following associations and organizations have been particularly fruitful: the American Public Health Association, the Food and Nutrition Section of the American Applied Economics Association, the Society for Nutrition Education and Behavior, the International Society for Behavioral Nutrition and Physical Activity, and the International Health Economics Association

We'd like to thank the administration at Virginia Tech for their recognition many years ago of the need to understand more about the intersection of food, nutrition, and economics and their commitment to supporting research and teaching in that area. We'd like to thank all our colleagues at Virginia Tech in the Departments of Human Nutrition, Foods, and Exercise and Agricultural and Applied Economics who have recognized the importance of this area of scholarship.

—GEORGE AND ELENA

Most of this book was written in 2014 while I was on sabbatical at Oxford University at the Centre of Time Use Research. I'd like to thank the Centre Directors, Jonathan Gershuny and Oriel Sullivan, for allowing me to be an academic visitor and Kimberly Fisher for graciously serving as my host. I would also like to express my gratitude to Donald Hay (retired economics professor from Jesus College) for numerous stimulating and educational conversations related to this book and many other topics. My productivity was greatly enhanced by the warm welcome I felt from Oxford and the community of Minster Lovell.

Closer to home, I want to especially thank my dear friend and colleague, Wen You, who has been a productive partner in much of the research related to this book. Of course my most important colleague in this project is my friend and coauthor Elena Serrano who has always been a joy to work with and has always shown good humor and patience with me in many ways, especially related to my nutrition questions. She has the mind of a true scholar, searching for truth wherever it may exist, be it in the field of nutrition, marketing, psychology, and yes even economics. Thanks Elena for being such a great colleague.

This book originated from notes used in a senior level course on Food and Nutrition Economics and I'd like to thank all of the students who have taken the course. The great feedback I have received from the students over the years greatly improved the book. I want to especially thank the former student Katie Caruthers who provided great assistance with checking the cited references and creating a reference database. The course and book also benefited from the great insights of three superb graduate teaching assistants over the years: Jackie Yenerall, Ranju Baral, and Yanliang Yang.

More personally, I want to thank the many friends who provided great encouragement while writing this book, especially those from Blacksburg Christian Fellowship Church. Most importantly, I want to thank the Lord and my family. My brothers Mac and Tony provided great encouragement and Tony read and provided editorial comments on the entire book. Finally, this book is dedicated to my lovely wife and daughter, Mellie and Olivia. Their support, encouragement, insights, prayers, and love sustained me on many a difficult day. Thank you and I love you. You were right, it could be finished!!

—GEORGE

I want to thank George for including me in this endeavor. It was his brain child and I'm honored to be part of it. I have appreciated George's dedication and commitment to this book in addition to his flexibility in answering countless questions about economics. The book has deep integrity, just like George, along with good humor. He is a fine person and good friend. I also want to thank: my original mentor and visionary, Jennifer Anderson, who had faith in me contributing to the nutrition field; all of my positive and supportive colleagues over the years, including Cindy Dallow, Kathy Hosig, Heather Boyd, and Mary McFerren; and, last but not least, all of my graduate students who constantly make me a better person and academic.

Thank you to my dear family who has provided constant support and love–especially my mother, my best friend, who has been by my side through thick and thin and who always knows I can do it, even when I don't; my amazing husband, Tod, who adds humor to everything; and my two boys who make me think about what my work and life means. I would also like to thank my friends, who help me be less serious. Finally, I credit lots of different pieces of my contribution here to both of my fathers.

—ELENA

Hello, everyone! My name is Jon Henry. I am Elena's 10-year old son. My brother is Paul Wyatt, who is eight. My mom decided to combine us into one person, a nutritionist, in the book, even though we give her a hard time about all of the healthy foods she offers us. In about 15 years we might even read the book in a course.

—JP

Hey folks! My name is Olivia Margaret Davis. I am George's 11 year old daughter. I was named for my Dad's mother. To pay homage to her and me, dad decided to use her name, Margaret, as the name of the economist is the book. I think you may actually enjoy the book as I can almost understand economics the way dad explains it!

—MARGARET

ABOUT THE AUTHORS

George C. Davis is an economics Professor at Virginia Tech. He holds a joint appointment in the Department of Human Nutrition, Foods, and Exercise and the Department of Agricultural and Applied Economics. His teaching and research programs both are interdisciplinary as he works with health scientists to understand issues at the intersection of nutrition, health, and economics.

Elena L. Serrano is a nutrition Associate Professor at Virginia Tech and the Director of the Virginia Family Nutrition Program aimed at promoting healthy eating among SNAP-eligible audiences throughout Virginia. Her research has focused on identifying and testing different programs, initiatives, and strategies to improve dietary quality and prevent childhood obesity among low-income youth, while incorporating economic principles within her framework.

PART I

An Introduction to Nutrition

This section of the book covers the basics of nutrition that are relevant for the economic analysis in the rest of the book. Chapter 1 covers the key concepts and definitions from nutrition and discusses the connection among nutrients, food, and health. Various metrics are presented and discussed for measuring nutrient intake. Dietary recommendations are covered as well as several nutrition information formats, such as the Nutrition Facts Label, MyPlate, and the Dietary Guidelines for Americans, which are designed to make following recommendations easier. Chapter 2 gives an overview of some of the data and trends in the United States on nutrient and food intake and diseases. Information is provided on what foods and nutrients are considered preventive in terms of some major chronic diseases.

PART 1

An Introduction to Nutrition

1

Food, Nutrients, and Health

AN OVERVIEW

Learning Objectives

What you will know by the end of this chapter:

- the complexity of understanding and applying nutrition;
- the relationship among nutrients, foods, and health;
- dietary recommendations and tools for healthy eating for the American public, including Dietary Reference Intakes, the Nutrition Facts Label, MyPlate, and the Dietary Guidelines for Americans;
- calculating nutrients within foods and meals;
- nutrition indices to quantify nutrition and dietary behaviors.

Opening Conversation

Setting: Standing in line at a coffee cart at a national multidisciplinary conference on Food, Nutrition, and Health, sponsored by the federal government

JP (to the barista): I will have a small cappuccino with nonfat milk. I would also like this apple.

Margaret: Wow! I was going to order a fancy drink with whipped cream. You chose something pretty healthy from all of these choices.

JP: Well, I am a nutritionist, so I try to practice what I preach, as the saying goes.

Margaret: So there is a job where you can tell people what to eat?

JP: Yes there is. That's exactly what I do. It's a really important area. With people so busy and on the run all the time, eating healthfully has become a lower priority. But it should be the top priority.

Margaret: As an economist, I try to avoid the word "should." I like whipped cream, for example, but I admit I do not know much about nutrition. I'd like to hear more about nutrition.

Background

Currently, chronic diseases affect approximately 117 million adults (49.8%) in the United States (Ward, Schiller, and Goodman 2014). Seven of the top 10 causes of death in the United States are *chronic diseases*, with heart disease and cancer alone accounting for almost half (46%) of all deaths (Centers for Disease Control and Prevention. National Center for Health Statistics 2014). See Table 1.1.

The economic consequences of chronic disease are astounding. According to a 2007 study, chronic diseases have a financial impact of $1.3 trillion annually; by 2023, this is estimated to increase to $4.2 trillion (DeVol and Bedroussian 2007;Wu and Green 2000). So, what role does nutrition play in chronic disease?

Nutrition

A person's *diet* or dietary behavior refers to what a person usually eats or drinks. Diet and dietary behaviors are important and significant factors in the prevention of chronic disease and the promotion of overall health. Together, over time, a person's dietary behavior informs the nutrition status of a person, which can range from poor to optimal. Optimal nutrition and healthy eating mean choosing foods that offer the optimal balance of nutrients for your body's needs, including quantities, proportions, variety, and combinations. Optimal nutrition lowers the risk for chronic disease, such as heart disease and cancer, the leading causes of death in the

TABLE 1.1

Leading Causes of Death in the United States Associated with Chronic Diseases[a]

Cause of Death	Number of Deaths (2012–2013)[b]
1. Heart disease	611,105
2. Cancer	584,881
3. Chronic lower respiratory diseases	149,205
4. Stroke	128,931
5. Accidents, unintentional injuries	130,557
6. Alzheimer's disease	84,767
7. Diabetes (type 1 and 2)	75,578
8. Influenza and pneumonia	56,979
9. Kidney disease	47,112
10. Suicide	41,149

[a] Shading denotes cause of death that is potentially attributed to food or nutrition factor.

[b] *Source:* Centers for Disease Control and Prevention, National Center for Health Statistics 2014.

United States. *Risk factors* are factors known to be related to (or correlated with) diseases but not proven to be causal.

WHAT ARE NUTRIENTS?

Every single food and beverage has a different nutrition profile with different nutrients that may be beneficial, or not. *Nutrients* are families of molecules in food—or components of food—that provide energy or assist with various mechanisms in the body's functioning. There are three major classes of nutrients: macronutrients (carbohydrates, protein, and fats, which are required in relatively large [macro] amounts); micronutrients (including vitamins and minerals, which are present and only needed in small, minute [micro] amounts); and water. Each type of nutrient has important and unique functions in addition to helping other nutrients function. *Macronutrients* are primarily responsible for providing your body with energy. They also have other functions, such as helping to maintain and repair the body. Alcohol also provides your body with energy, but it is not considered a macronutrient since it is not needed for survival. Energy is measured in *kilocalories*, the amount of energy needed to raise the temperature of one kilogram of water by one degree Celsius. In nutrition, such as on menus or food packages, kilocalories is shortened to simply "calorie." Calories often serve as a guide for weight management. Each person requires a certain amount of calories for the body to function, based on age, gender, and physical activity level. As a result, if you consume more calories than your body requires, you can gain weight. *Micronutrients* do not provide energy but assist with a wide range of other functions within the body, such as helping to utilize the macronutrients and building bones, teeth, and muscles, depending on the actual micronutrient. As you will see by reviewing all of the macro- and micronutrients, not one nutrient can meet all of the body's needs. As a result, your diet should comprise a wide variety of foods.

MACRONUTRIENTS

Of the macronutrients, *carbohydrates* are compounds that are composed of either single or multiple sugars. They are classified by the number of sugar units they contain. The higher number of units, the longer it takes your body to break it down and process. Sugar (sucrose) that you add to coffee or tea has only two units. Each type of sugar has different attributes. Complex carbohydrates have multiple units and are mainly found in starchy foods like grains, such as (wheat) flour (used to make bread and flour tortillas), potatoes, and rice. They can be found in other foods, but in smaller amounts. There are 4 calories per each gram of carbohydrate. *Fats and oils* are organic compounds that are soluble in organic solvents (lipids) but not in water. They are made of fatty acids and glycerol. Fats, such as butter, shortening, and bacon fat, are solid at room temperature. Oils, such as olive oil and corn oil, are liquid. They are further classified as saturated fatty acids, usually solid, and unsaturated (mono- and poly-) fatty acids, generally liquid. The properties and effects are different because of their structure. Fats and oils will be described simply as "fats" in the remainder of the book, unless noted. Unsaturated fatty acids are preferred over saturated or solid fatty acids. There are 9 calories per gram of fat. In addition to offering more than twice the amount of calories per gram, fat also helps with the absorption of certain vitamins. *Proteins* are organic compounds composed of chains of amino acids joined by peptide bonds. Good sources of protein include dried beans and meat. Like carbohydrates, there are 4 calories per gram of protein. Protein is associated with building and repair of tissues and muscles.

MICRONUTRIENTS

Vitamins are organic compounds that regulate the chemical processes that take place in the body. There are 13 indispensable vitamins for body functions: vitamin A, vitamin C, vitamin D, vitamin E, vitamin K, and the B vitamins (thiamine, riboflavin, niacin, pantothenic acid, biotin, vitamin B-6, vitamin B-12, and folate). There are two groups of vitamins, depending on how they are carried in food and transported in the body: water-soluble vitamins and fat-soluble vitamins. Water-soluble vitamins are not stored in the body after they are utilized; they are excreted through your urine. Fat-soluble vitamins are stored in the body and dissolved in fat. This distinction is important because consuming or taking too many of some fat-soluble vitamins can be harmful in some cases. *Minerals* are naturally occurring inorganic substances or chemical elements. They cannot be destroyed by heat, such as when cooking. Like vitamins, there are also numerous essential minerals. They assist with vitamins and also help with body maintenance and forming new tissue, like bones, teeth, and blood. There are macro (or major) minerals and trace minerals, depending on how much you need. We will focus on the ones of biggest public health concern. Calcium, phosphorus, magnesium, sodium, potassium, chloride, and sulfur are macro minerals, and iron, manganese, copper, iodine, zinc, cobalt, fluoride, and selenium are trace minerals. Foods can contain micro- and macronutrients. For example, ground beef (used to make hamburgers) contains protein (macronutrient), fat (macronutrient; amount depends on how lean the meat is), vitamin B-12 (vitamin), and zinc (mineral).

FIBER

Although not considered a nutrient per se, dietary fiber is an integral component of plant structure. It is considered nondigestible and offers physiological benefits, such as improving intestinal health and helping to prevent heart disease and some cancers.

WATER

Approximately two-thirds of our body weight is made up of water. It helps carry nutrients and oxygen to cells. It helps make minerals and other nutrients accessible to the body. It also is used to remove waste products from the body. In addition to low-fat milk, water is the best choice of beverage.

ALCOHOL

Alcohol is not considered a macronutrient, although it is a fermented product of carbohydrates, because it is not required. It is not even considered a nutrient; however, it is energy producing and supplies 7 calories per gram and is a major source of calories in many individuals.

Connection Among Nutrients, Food, and Health

Table 1.2 shows the different macro- and micronutrients, some of their general functions, and popular food sources of each nutrient, in addition to fiber. As you can see, nutrients can be found across different types and groups of foods either naturally or by being added (e.g., fortified).

For example, vitamin E can be found in wheat germ, nuts and seeds, vegetable oils, and even fruit. That also means, as we mentioned earlier, that most foods and beverages contain more than one nutrient, although they may be a good source of one or two in particular. For example, low-fat milk contains protein, carbohydrate, fat, calcium, vitamin D, and negligible amounts of other vitamins and minerals. As a result, eating a variety of foods each day and over time is important to ensure the intake of a well-balanced portfolio of nutrients.

Dietary Recommendations

DIETARY REFERENCE INTAKES: REFERENCE NUTRIENT VALUES

What we have presented about nutrition so far probably seems pretty straightforward. However, applying this information daily can become complicated. The *Dietary Reference Intakes* (DRIs) were created to help provide specific values for specific nutrients for optimal health, as well as values that should not be exceeded (U.S. Department of Agriculture, National Agricultural Library 2015). The DRIs are shown in the last two columns of Table 1.2 for each key nutrient for females and males 19 to 30 years old. (There are DRIs for other age groups and for pregnant women, but these were chosen for reference.) DRIs are developed and updated by the National Academy of Sciences' Institute of Medicine's Food and Nutrition Board based on scientific evidence. DRIs are assigned for all of the vitamins and minerals, as well as carbohydrates, fiber, lipids, protein, water, and calories. DRI is an umbrella term that refers to four sets of reference nutrient values, depending on the extent of research to support or not support a recommendation for a nutrient.

TABLE 1.2
Key Nutrients in Health Promotion and Disease Prevention

Class of Nutrient	Specific Nutrient	Function	Most Common Food Source(s)	Primary Food Group(s) of MyPlate	Notes about the Guidelines	Dietary Recommended Intakes (DRIs)[a] Females 19-30 y	Males 19-30 y
Macronutrient	Carbohydrates	Primary energy source for the brain	Complex carbohydrates ◻ Bread ◻ Pasta ◻ Potatoes ◻ Rice ◻ Vegetables Simple sugars ◻ Naturally in fruit ◻ Added to sodas/soft drinks, fruit drinks, desserts, and candy	Grains	Individuals should limit the amount of added sugars in their diets. Fruits, with naturally occurring sugars, are considered beneficial because of the vitamins, minerals, and fiber they contain regardless of the sugar content (assuming no sugar is added like syrup).	130 g/day (RDA/AI) 45–65% of total calories (ADMR) <10% of total calories from added sugar[b]	130 g/day (RDA/AI) 45–65% of total calories (ADMR) <10% of total calories from added sugar[b]
Macronutrient	Fat	Energy source and energy storage Also helps with absorption of fat-soluble vitamins (e.g., vitamin A)	◻ Butter ◻ Margarine ◻ Vegetable oil ◻ Grain-based desserts (cookies, cake, pie) ◻ Pizza ◻ Cheese ◻ Fatty meats like sausages and bacon ◻ French fries	Naturally in protein (fatty sources of animal protein) and dairy (unless nonfat or low-fat), but can be added to foods in all food groups	Trans fats and saturated fats, generally fats solid at room temperature, should be limited. They are present in animal fats (e.g., sausages and fat), coconut oil, and palm kernel oil. Oils that are high in omega-3 (ω-3) fatty acids are considered beneficial and healthy fats. These include olive oils, fatty fish, and oil found in nuts and seeds.	20–35% of total calories (ADMR) <10% of total calories from saturated fat[b]	20–35% of total calories (ADMR) <10% of total calories from saturated fat[b]

(continued)

Macronutrient				46 g/day	56 g/day
Protein and amino acids (building blocks of protein)	Provide structure to the body Function as enzymes and sometimes hormones	Animal sources ¤ Beef ¤ Pork ¤ Chicken ¤ Fish ¤ Eggs ¤ Dairy products Vegetable sources ¤ Dried beans/ legumes ¤ Grains ¤ Seeds ¤ Nuts	Protein	Nine amino acids are called "essential" and must be provided in the diet. The body can synthesize the other specific amino acids. Proteins from animal sources are considered "complete." Vegetable proteins, from plants, dried beans/legumes, nuts, and seeds, are considered "incomplete" and must be combined to form a "complete" protein.	
Vitamin (Essential 13)				700 µg/day (RDA)	900 µg/day (RDA)
Vitamin A *Fat-soluble*	Night vision and prevention of disease	¤ Brightly colored fruits ¤ Leafy green vegetables ¤ Meat ¤ Dairy products ¤ Fortified ready-to-eat cereals (read the Nutrition Facts Label)	Fruits and vegetables	There are two types of vitamin A: preformed found in meat and dairy, and pro-vitamin A in produce. Excessive amounts of preformed vitamin A, usually in the form of vitamin supplements, in pregnant women can cause birth defects in their babies.	

TABLE 1.2
Continued

Class of Nutrient	Specific Nutrient	Function	Most Common Food Source(s)	Primary Food Group(s) of MyPlate	Notes about the Guidelines	Dietary Recommended Intakes (DRIs)[a]	
						Females 19–30 y	Males 19–30 y
Vitamin	Vitamin B-1 (thiamine, aneurin), vitamin B-2 (riboflavin), vitamin B-3 (niacin), vitamin B-5 (pantothenic acid), vitamin B-6 (pyridoxal, pyridoxine, pyridoxamine), vitamin B-12 (cobalamin), folate (folic acid) *Water-soluble*	Help with energy utilization	◻ Meat ◻ Fish ◻ Dairy products ◻ Dried beans/legumes ◻ Fortified ready-to-eat cereals ◻ Whole-grain products ◻ Bread and bread products	Grains	The B vitamins are often classified together, since they have similar functions and can be found in similar foods. The lack of B-6 and B-12 can cause anemia.	B-1, B-2: 1.1 mg/day B-3: 14 mg/day B-6: 1.3 mg/day B-12: 2.4 µg/day Folate: 400 µg/day (RDA)	B-1: 1.2 mg/day B-2: 1.3 mg/day B-3: 14 mg/day B-6: 1.3 mg/day B-12: 2.4 µg/day Folate: 400 µg/day (RDA)
Vitamin	Vitamin C (ascorbic acid) *Water-soluble*	Heals wounds, builds connective tissue, helps with iron absorption	◻ Citrus fruits ◻ Tomatoes ◻ Brussels sprouts ◻ Cauliflower ◻ Broccoli ◻ Sweet potatoes ◻ Spinach	Fruits and vegetables		75 mg/day (RDA)	90 mg/day (RDA)
Vitamin	Vitamin D (calciferol) *Fat-soluble*	Assists with calcium absorption and promotes bone health	◻ Fortified dairy ◻ Bread and grain products ◻ Sunshine (when ultraviolet rays from sunlight hit the skin, vitamin D is made)	Dairy	It is naturally present in very few foods.	15 µg/day (RDA)	15 µg/day (RDA)

Type	Nutrient	Function	Food Sources	Food Group	Notes		
Vitamin	Vitamin E (α-tocopherol) *Fat-soluble*	Protects tissues from oxidation	¤ Wheat germ ¤ Nuts and seeds ¤ Vegetable oils ¤ Fruit	Grains and protein		15 mg/day (RDA)	15 mg/day (RDA)
Vitamin	Vitamin K (derived from German word *koagulation*) *Fat-soluble*	Helps with the function and synthesis of many proteins involved in blood clotting and bone metabolism	¤ Green leafy vegetables (collards, kale, spinach, Swiss chard, salad greens, broccoli) ¤ Dark berries ¤ Vegetable oils and margarine	Vegetables	Vitamin K can also be made in the body.	90 µg/day (AI)	120 µg/day (AI)
Mineral (Select)	Calcium	Bone and tooth formation, role in blood clotting and nerve transmission	¤ Dairy products ¤ Corn tortillas ¤ Calcium-fortified tofu ¤ Chinese cabbage ¤ Kale ¤ Broccoli ¤ Calcium-fortified foods and beverages (e.g., orange juice, soy milk)	Dairy		1000 mg/day (RDA)	1000 mg/day (RDA)
Mineral	Iron	Helps build red blood cells along with protein to carry oxygen throughout the body	¤ Meat ¤ Fortified bread and grain products ¤ Fruits ¤ Vegetables	Protein	Meat sources contain heme iron, which is more readily absorbed by the body. Lack of iron can lead to anemia.	18 mg/day (RDA)	8 mg/day (RDA)
Mineral	Magnesium	Aids in production of energy; helps muscles, arteries, and heart function properly	¤ Vegetables ¤ Wheat bran ¤ Nuts	Vegetables		310 mg/day (RDA)	400 mg/day (RDA)

(continued)

TABLE 1.2
Continued

Class of Nutrient	Specific Nutrient	Function	Most Common Food Source(s)	Primary Food Group(s) of MyPlate	Notes about the Guidelines	Dietary Recommended Intakes (DRIs)[a]	
						Females 19-30 y	Males 19-30 y
Mineral	Potassium	Helps muscles contract and nerves communicate; aids in regulation of blood pressure	¤ Leafy greens (spinach and collard greens) ¤ Fruit from vines like blackberries and grapes ¤ Root vegetables (carrots, potatoes) ¤ Dairy products	Vegetables		4.7 g/day (AI)	4.7 g/day (AI)
Mineral	Sodium	Maintains fluid volume and blood pressure, assists with muscle and nerve function	¤ Salt ¤ Processed foods such as bread, cheese, pizza, cold cuts, and snacks like potato chips, pretzels, and crackers	Protein		2,300 mg/day[b]	2,300 mg/day[b]
Mineral	Zinc	Helps the immune system (fighting infection, wound healing), synthesizes proteins and DNA Involved in gene regulation Considered an immune promoter	¤ Red meats ¤ Certain seafood and fish ¤ Fortified ready-to-eat cereals	Protein, Fruits, vegetables, and (whole) grains		8 mg/day (RDA)	11 mg/day (RDA)

Other	Fiber	Aids with digestive health	✷ Whole grains (oats, wheat, unmilled rice, etc.) ✷ Fresh fruits ✷ Fresh vegetables	Fruits, vegetables, and (whole) grains		25 g/day (AI)	38 g/day (AI)
Other	Water	Helps transport nutrients and oxygen to cells	✷ All water contained in food, beverages, and drinking water	Water		2.7 l/day	3.7 l/day
Other	Alcohol	Relaxant	✷ Beer, wine, distilled spirits (hard alcohol)	Not included in MyPlate		Up to one drink per day[d]	Up to two drinks per day[d]
Other	Calories (kcal)	Needed to generate energy for body functions and movement	✷ All foods, many beverages (except water and artificially sweetened beverages)	Across all food groups	Kilocalories is often expressed in kilojoules (kJ): 1 kcal = 4.184 kJ	2,100 kcal/day[e]	2,700 kcal/day[e]

[a] U.S. Department of Agriculture, National Agricultural Library 2015. View recommended intake tables for the complete list of DRIs for all nutrients and age groups.

[b] Based on the 2015 Dietary Guidelines for Americans. U.S. Department of Health and Human Services 2015.

[c] The DGAs recommend limiting sodium to less than 2,300 mg/day. Some individuals may need to limit sodium to 1,500 mg/day.

[d] Based on the 2010 DGAs, only for adults of legal drinking age. One drink is 12 fluid ounces of regular beer (5% alcohol), 5 fluid ounces of wine (12% alcohol), or 1.5 fluid ounces of 80 proof (40% alcohol) distilled spirits. One drink contains 0.6 fluid ounces of alcohol. U.S. Department of Health and Human Services 2010.

[e] Based on the USDA Center for Nutrition Policy Promotion using averages for age groups within this range by gender and for moderately active individuals. U.S. Department of Health and Human Services 2010, Appendix 6.

Note: AMDR: Acceptable Macronutrient Distribution Range. It is the range of intake for macronutrients that is ensures adequate essential nutrients and a reduced risk of chronic disease.

◻ *Estimated Average Requirement (EAR)*—The average daily intake level for a nutrient that meets the needs of 50% of the population in particular life stages and gender groups.

◻ *Recommended Dietary Allowance (RDA)*—The average daily nutrient intake level that meets the needs of nearly all (97–98%) healthy people in a particular life stage and gender group.

◻ *Adequate Intake (AI)*—The recommended average daily nutrient intake levels based on intakes of healthy people (observed or experimentally derived) in a particular life stage and gender group and assumed to be adequate. This is usually assigned when there is not enough evidence for an RDA.

◻ *Tolerable Upper Intake Levels (ULs)*—The highest average daily nutrient intake level that is likely to pose no risk of toxicity to almost all healthy individuals of a particular life stage and gender group.

Consumers can see the DRIs in use on the Nutrition Facts Label of food products (which we review later in this chapter) and on vitamin and mineral supplements.

Nutrition Metrics

So far, we have reviewed several important concepts about nutrition: (1) Nutrition is determined by what foods and beverages a person consumes and what nutrients are in those foods and beverages; (2) Each nutrient is unique in what it offers the body; and (3) the DRIs provide specific recommendations or thresholds for each nutrient for different ages and gender to reach optimal nutrition.

But how do you know if you are actually meeting the DRI for a specific nutrient? How do you make the "best" food and beverage choices to meet all of the DRIs? How do you determine which nutrient(s) to be concerned about? What changes could you make in individual food choices, meal choices, or your overall diet to improve your overall nutrition? There are so many different nutrients and even more foods and beverages. We are not even mentioning what you like to eat or economic constraints, such as how much money you have to spend on food.

CALCULATING THE AMOUNT OF NUTRIENTS
AND CALORIES IN INDIVIDUAL FOODS

Here we will begin to see how quantifying nutrients can be used to meet target DRIs within different food choice and nutrition scenarios. What you will find over and over is that nutrition is about balancing the choice of foods (and quantities of foods), macronutrients, and micronutrients.

Since all foods, with the exception of water (and many beverages that use artificial sweeteners), contain calories (kilocalories) and calories are a simple metric for determining if a person is eating too much or too little, let's begin by using a formula to calculate the amount of calories in a food. Remember, each gram of carbohydrate and protein yields 4 calories and each gram of fat 9 calories. So, the amount of calories (kcals, cals) in a food is determined by the equation:

$$Total\ Calories = (4\ cals/gram \times Carbohydrates\ in\ grams)$$
$$+ (4\ cals/gram \times Protein\ in\ grams)$$
$$+ (9\ cals/gram \times Fat\ in\ grams)$$

This equation can also be shown more simply using variable notation, which is used throughout this book.

$$kcals = 4 \times N_C + 4 \times N_P + 9 \times N_F \qquad (1.1)$$

where:

$kcals$ = calories (kcal) in grams,
N_C = carbohydrates in grams,
N_P = protein in grams,
N_F = fat in grams.

What does this look like for an actual food or beverage? If a food has 40 grams of carbohydrates (N_C = 40), 30 grams of protein (N_P = 30), and 20 grams of fat (N_F = 20) then inserting into Equation 1.1 we obtain: 460 calories = (4 × 40) + (4 × 30) + (9 × 20). And yes, most units in nutrition are in grams.

As you can see from this equation, there are different ways you can influence total calories, depending on how much of each macronutrient is in a food or beverage. This means that there are *substitution* possibilities. If you replace or substitute one macronutrient, for example protein, with another, such as fat, which contains more than twice the amount of calories per gram, you can change the total number of calories. Alternatively, you can change the amount of nutrients while keeping the calories the same or constant. For example, since carbohydrates and protein contain the same number of calories per gram (4), if you decrease carbohydrates by one gram and increase protein by one gram, the calories would not change. In this case, this would be considered an isocalorie substitution. Both examples demonstrate that there are *trade-offs* among carbohydrates, fats, and protein.

Now, let's see what this looks like with popular fast food foods and beverages (Table 1.3). Using Equation 1.1, the total number of calories for the Big Mac hamburger is 590 cals = (4 × 47) + (4 × 24) + (9 × 34). The other foods and beverages are calculated the same way. Note that the chicken has almost the same number of calories (610 cals) as the Big Mac but for different reasons. Whereas the Big Mac has 47 grams of carbohydrates, the chicken has only 21 grams. Alternatively, the chicken has 54 grams of protein whereas the Big Mac has 24. This example

TABLE 1.3
Nutritional Characteristics of Select Food Items[a]

Food Item	Quantity	Weight (g)	Carbohydrates (g)	Protein (g)	Fat (g)	Energy (cals)
McDonald's Big Mac* (hamburger)	1 item	216	47	24	34	590
Side salad (no dressing)	1 small	87	4	1	0	20
Coca-Cola Classic	12 oz	360	39	0	0	156
KFC Original Recipe* chicken breast and thigh	1 item	288	21	54	35	615

[a] Sources: McDonalds 2014, Kentucky Fried Chicken 2014.

demonstrates that similar calorie levels do not mean they have the same macronutrient composition. They will not have the exact micronutrient or fiber composition either.

Taking this further to include micronutrients, consider two other examples (U.S. Department of Agriculture, Agricultural Research Service 2014):

- One container of nonfat (fat-free), fruit-flavored yogurt (8 ounces): 216 calories; 10 grams of protein; 0.45 grams of fat (of which 0.3 grams is saturated); 43 grams of carbohydrate; and 202 mg of calcium
- Two slices of cheddar cheese (2 ounces): 227 calories; 13.5 grams of protein; 19 grams of fat (10.8 grams saturated fat); 0.74 grams of carbohydrate; and 378 mg of calcium

Which one would be best if you were trying to limit saturated fat? Which one would be best if you wanted to maximize calcium? What about if both were important to you?

CALCULATING THE AMOUNT OF NUTRIENTS AND CALORIES IN MEALS

With the exception of newborns, individuals usually do not eat just one individual food. Instead, people eat several foods at a time as part of a meal or snack. Still, the same calculations can be applied to a meal. Suppose Meal 1 consists of a Big Mac, a side salad, and a 12-ounce Coca-Cola and Meal 2 consists of two pieces of fried chicken, a side salad, and a 12-ounce Coca-Cola.

For Meal 1 the total weight is 663 g = 216 g + 87 g + 360 g. The total grams of carbohydrate is 90 g = 47 g + 4 g + 39 g, total protein is 25 g = 24 g + 1 g, and total fat is 34 g = 34 g + 0 g + 0 g. Using Equation 1.1, the total calories for Meal 1 is 766 = (4 × 90) + (4 × 25) + (9 × 34). The same procedure would apply to Meal 2, resulting in 735 grams of weight, 64 grams carbohydrate, 55 grams protein, 35 grams fat, and 791 total calories. While the total calories of the two meals are similar, the distribution of the calories across the macronutrients is very different, mostly because of the carbohydrate and protein profiles. The total amount of fat is similar, however. So, if you wanted to make a decision based on total fat, neither would be a necessarily better option (especially since they represent about half of total fat needed based on a 2,000-kcal diet). The choice would depend on which is more important—carbohydrate, protein, or another nutrient.

CALCULATING THE AMOUNT OF NUTRIENTS AND CALORIES IN A DIET

We have reviewed how to compare calories (only one factor in nutrition) for individual foods and even meals. Now, how do we calculate the amount of nutrients over the course of a day, week, or longer? The same type of approach can be used. One way to do this is to use the *nutrient conversion factor*, a multiplier that converts the number of grams in a food to the amount of the nutrient in the food in grams. Consider foods as bundles of nutrients or a delivery device for nutrients.

We can use the Big Mac meal as an example. There are 47 g of carbohydrates in a Big Mac hamburger that weighs 216 g. This means that $0.218 = 47/216$ of the total grams in a Big Mac hamburger are associated with carbohydrates. The carbohydrate conversion factor for this food is 0.218. The carbohydrate conversion factor is $0.0460 = 4/87$ for salad and $0.108 = 39/360$ for Coca-Cola. For Meal 1 (Big Mac, side salad, and a 12-ounce Coca-Cola Classic), the conversion factors for carbohydrates are 0.218, 0.0460, and 0.108. The total carbohydrates for Meal 1 is then $90 = 0.218 \times 216 + 0.0460 \times 87 + 0.108 \times 360$. The nutrient conversion factor gives you the nutrients per gram, so if you ate more and the number of grams consumed changed, you simply multiply by the nutrient conversion factor to get the new quantity of the nutrient. You would not need to stop at just the meal, however. You could add other foods and beverages you consumed over the course of a day, week, and so forth.

The general formula for doing this is:

$$N_j = \alpha_{j1}F_1 + \alpha_{j2}F_2 + ... + \alpha_{jK}F_K \quad j = 1, 2, ..., J \tag{1.2}$$

where there are J nutrients.

Variable F_1 denotes the quantity (in grams) of the first food item, F_2 denotes the quantity (in grams) of the second food item, F_3 the quantity (in grams) of the third food item, and so forth, or more generally F_k where k is just an indexing mechanism and $k = 1, 2, \ldots, K$ so there are K foods. Furthermore let α_{11} be the nutrient conversion factor for Nutrient 1 in Food 1, α_{12} be the nutrient conversion factor for Nutrient 1 in Food 2, α_{13} be the nutrient conversion factor for Nutrient 1 in Food 3, and so forth. The j subscript on the nutrient conversion factors is to show that the nutrient conversion factors differ by nutrient and food item.

It goes now without saying that you can use this formula to also determine the micronutrients across the foods and beverages you eat. For example, suppose you have eaten an orange for breakfast and a banana for lunch and you want to know how much vitamin C you obtained from these two fruits. A typical banana weighs about 120 grams and a typical orange weighs about 130 grams. Furthermore, there are about 0.01 and 0.07 grams of vitamin C in a banana and an orange, respectively (U.S. Department of Agriculture, Agricultural Research Service 2014). Or, in terms of the nutrient conversion factors of vitamins per gram, there are 0.000083 grams of vitamin C per gram of a banana and 0.00054 grams of vitamin C per gram of an orange. Using Equation 1.2, then, the amount of vitamin C from these two fruits is 0.08 g = 0.000083 × 120 + 0.00054 × 130 = 0.01 + 0.07 or 80 mg. You can then compare these to how much you need per day. How are you doing? (Hint: See Table 1.2)

Notice what is required for these calculations. You must first know the nutrient conversion factor in each food item, then you must multiply this times the amount of the food item eaten, and finally you must add these values up across all food items containing that nutrient. Calculating the total amount of nutrients from a set of foods in this manner can help you compare nutrition attributes of different choices.

Is your head hurting yet? If so, you are not alone. And it's OK. These equations and calculations are admittedly difficult. They are also not feasible for most consumers to compute when making daily decisions about food and nutrition. As a result, dietary and nutrition recommendations use several different formats and approaches to appeal to and inform the public. These range from food-based guides to mostly textual information that link DRIs and specific nutrition recommendations to health.

Foundation of Food and Nutrition–Based Guidelines

THE NUTRITION FACTS LABEL: A FOOD AND NUTRITION–BASED GUIDE

A tool to assist consumers with linking food with nutrients is the Nutrition Facts Label, found on most food and beverage products (U.S. Food and Drug Administration 2015a).[1] The Nutrition Facts Label contains specific nutrition information for food and beverage products to show how much of key nutrients are found in each food and beverage. It can also be used to compare the nutritional profile of different products. Since there is limited space on food products, the label contains nutrition information only for nutrients of public health concern, such as sodium, added sugars, saturated fat, vitamin D, potassium, and iron. It also contains information on macronutrients (fat, carbohydrates ["carbs"], and protein) and calories (Fig. 1.1).

Daily values (DVs) are used to help individuals relate the nutrition information in the product to what they need for a whole day for nutrients with established

[1] You may ask which ones don't have labels: fresh fruits and vegetables found in the produce section; foods produced by a company with fewer than 50 employees (such as what you might find at the farmers' market); and alcohol, since it's not under the administration of the U.S. Food and Drug Administration.

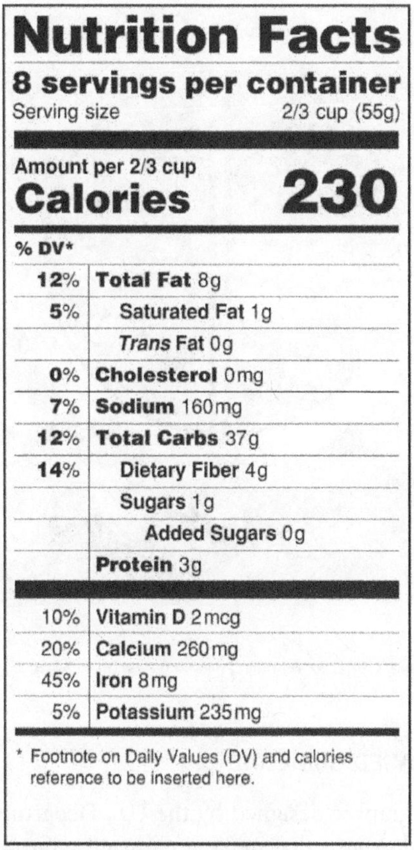

Nutrition Facts

8 servings per container

Serving size   2/3 cup (55g)

Amount per 2/3 cup

Calories   230

% DV*

12%	**Total Fat** 8g
5%	Saturated Fat 1g
	Trans Fat 0g
0%	**Cholesterol** 0mg
7%	**Sodium** 160mg
12%	**Total Carbs** 37g
14%	Dietary Fiber 4g
	Sugars 1g
	Added Sugars 0g
	Protein 3g
10%	Vitamin D 2mcg
20%	Calcium 260mg
45%	Iron 8mg
5%	Potassium 235mg

* Footnote on Daily Values (DV) and calories reference to be inserted here.

FIGURE 1.1 Nutrition Facts Label[a]

[a] U.S. Food and Drug Administration 2015b. This is based on the proposed changes to the Nutrition Facts Label, as of December 19, 2015. The percent daily value (%DV) tells you how much a nutrient is a serving of food contributes to a daily diet. 2,000 calories a day is used for general nutrition advice.

DRIs. The daily values are *daily* nutrient standards expressed as a percentage of a 2,000-calorie diet. (Suggestion: Look at Table 1.2 to see who 2,000 calories are appropriate for.) The DVs are actually calculated using the levels present in the food package divided by the DRI for that nutrient.

Some DVs are intended to help consumers limit intake, such as sodium and saturated fat, and others are to help meet the recommendation, such as potassium and vitamin D. (Why isn't there a DV for added sugars? Hint: Look at Table 1.2 to see the DRI.) The general rule of thumb is that 5% is considered low and 20% high. Based on the example in Figure 1.1, the product contains 260 mg of calcium, equating to 20% of the DV (based on a 2,000-calorie diet), meaning it would be considered a good source of calcium. It also contains only one gram of saturated fat, 5% of the daily recommendation, so it would be considered low in saturated fat.

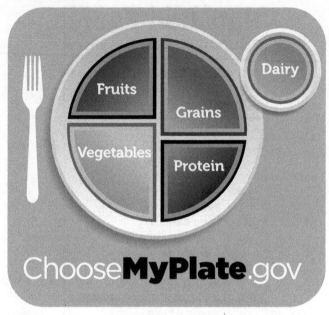

FIGURE 1.2 MyPlate[a]

[a] U.S. Department of Agriculture, Center for Nutrition Policy and Promotion 2014.

MYPLATE: A FOOD-BASED GUIDELINE

MyPlate is a simple graphic designed by the U.S. Department of Agriculture to show foods and food groups that make up a healthy meal (U.S. Department of Agriculture, Center for Nutrition Policy and Promotion 2014). MyPlate illustrates the five food groups that are the building blocks for a healthy diet, also shown in Table 1.2, using a familiar image—a place setting for a meal (Fig. 1.2).

As shown, half of the plate should comprise fruits and vegetables, with proportionally more vegetables than fruit. Grains (carbohydrates: breads, ready-to-eat cereals, pasta, rice, etc.) and protein (meat and dried beans/legumes) should fill the other half of the plate, with less protein than grains. Fat-free or low-fat milk or other calcium-rich foods should be offered with every meal as well.

MyPlate reinforces the concept that individuals eat food, not necessarily nutrients, although the food groups and proportions are based upon the DRIs. If you eat meals and snacks according to MyPlate, you will achieve the nutritional targets and recommendations for all macro- and micronutrients, and you won't require nutritional supplements.

THE DIETARY GUIDELINES FOR AMERICANS: FOOD, NUTRITION, AND HEALTH–BASED GUIDELINE

Finally, the Dietary Guidelines for Americans (DGAs) are a set of broad nutrition (and physical activity, although we will not review these in this book)

TABLE 1.4

Relationship Among Foods, Nutrition, and Health[a]

Dietary or Eating Behavior	Health Condition or Disease
Consumption of large portion sizes	Association with higher body weight
A diet high in fruits, vegetables, whole grains, nuts, dried beans/legumes, low-fat dairy, poultry, and fish; low in red and processed meat, high-fat dairy, and sugar-sweetened foods and beverages; and moderate in alcohol	Decreased risk of heart disease and stroke
High frequency of eating food from fast-food restaurants	Increased risk of weight gain, overweight, and obesity in children and adults
Consumption of diet aligned with DASH (Dietary Approaches to Stop Hypertension) diet—rich in fruits, vegetables, low-fat dairy, fish, whole grains, fiber, potassium, and other minerals and low in red and processed meat, sugar-sweetened foods and drinks, saturated fat, cholesterol, and sodium	Reduced blood pressure
High intake of saturated fat	Increased risk of heart disease and type 2 diabetes
High intake of mono-unsaturated fatty acids (MUFA)	Better blood cholesterol levels related to heart disease and diabetes
Replacement of saturated and trans fatty acids with poly-unsaturated fatty acids (PUFA)	Lower risk of heart disease and type 2 diabetes
Decrease in sodium intake	Decrease in blood pressure in adults
High intake of sugar-sweetened beverages (e.g., soft drinks, soda, fruit drinks)	Increased adiposity (body fat) in children
Control of caloric intake, regardless of proportion of carbohydrate, protein, and fat intake	Weight loss
Folate supplementation	No change in heart disease risk
Increase in potassium intake	Lower heart disease risk
Decrease in sodium intake	Lower blood pressure
Self-monitoring of food intake	Improved diet

[a] Based on "strong" evidence by the U.S. Department of Agriculture, Nutrition Evidence Library 2014. See dietary patterns full report.

recommendations and strategies for all individuals (U.S. Department of Health and Human Services 2010 and 2015).[2] The DGAs are based on a summary and synthesis of scientific research and knowledge about individual nutrients and food components and their relationship to health, including the DRIs. Table 1.4 shows the food, nutrition, and health connections that were rated "strong," based on the strength and integrity of the studies and other criteria. The overall body of evidence

---

[2] The DGAs are required to be updated every five years. The DGAs for 2015–2020 were released. They can be found at: http://health.gov/dietaryguidelines/2015/guidelines/.

identifies that a healthy dietary pattern is higher in vegetables, fruits, whole grains, low-fat or nonfat dairy, seafood, legumes, and nuts; moderate in alcohol (among adults); lower in red and processed meats; and low in sugar-sweetened foods and drinks and refined grains.

The DGAs are generally used more by professionals than by actual consumers. Still, they act as a framework for local, state, and national health-promotion and chronic-disease–prevention programs and initiatives, such as many nutrition assistance programs sponsored by the U.S. government, including the Special Supplemental Nutrition Program for Women, Infants, and Children (U.S. Department of Agriculture, Food and Nutrition Service, WIC 2015b), the Expanded Food and Nutrition Education Program (U.S. Department of Agriculture, National Institute of Food and Agriculture, EFNEP 2015), and the Supplemental Nutrition Assistance Program Education (U.S. Department of Agriculture, Food and Nutrition Service, SNAP-Ed 2015), some of which we will cover in this book.

FOOD FOR THOUGHT

If you think of the different food and nutrition guides as different components of building a house, the DGAs are the foundation and the framing of the house. The DGAs make sure that the house (health) is structurally sound and safe (nutrients). MyPlate is an image of the final completed house, which could not be possible without the DGAs. And the Nutrition Facts Label is like a blueprint of the house with legends assigned to only a few features of the house.

Let's do a simple example with calcium to show the differences between the different food and nutrition guidance tools.[3]

¤ The Scientific Report of the 2015 DGAs considers calcium as a nutrient of public health concern because "underconsumption has been linked in the scientific literature to adverse health outcomes" (U.S. Department of Health and Human Services 2015, p. 2). The 2010 DGAs recommend increasing intake of fat-free or low-fat milk and milk products, such as milk, yogurt, cheese, or fortified soy beverages, based on evidence that calcium status is important for bone health (U.S. Department of Health and Human Services 2010).
¤ The RDA for calcium for males and females is 1,000 mg per day. If one standard portion of nonfat milk contains approximately 300 mg of calcium, roughly how many servings in a day would you need?

---

[3] You can also find the quantity of a nutrient in any food product by searching the online U.S. Department of Agriculture, Agricultural Research Service 2014 database.

¤ What foods and beverages contain calcium? Where are they found in MyPlate? How might you balance your plate to ensure that you obtain enough calcium?

¤ If the Nutrition Facts Label stated that a product contained 10% of the calcium RDA, how many servings would you require in a day to meet this recommendation? (Additionally, is this a "good" source of calcium?) Or what other food or beverage choices could you make to get enough calcium?

Nutrition Indices

There are a lot of things to think about when you are making a food choice with nutrition in mind. So many nutrients, all in different combinations in foods, with many trade-offs! It seems like there should be a way to summarize and/or rate a food or a diet by a single number. There is! There are several terms for it, including nutrition indices, nutrition rating systems, or nutrient profiling systems or models. They all aim to do essentially the same thing—simplify food choices. A *nutrition index* is an equation that categorizes foods and/or diets for the purpose of health, based on their nutritional characteristics. In other words, it allows for ranking of foods and diets based on their nutrient content. Other approaches expand on this concept to encompass all nutrients and, if desired, all foods that someone eats as part of his or her diet. Indices have become increasingly popular on different food packages to inform consumers of the nutritional value of the product. They have also been used by manufacturers and even national policy in the United Kingdom to guide sales and legislation regulating food advertising to children, respectively.

The challenge really becomes what to include in the equation. Should the index include all nutrients or just selected nutrients? If select nutrients, should it focus on "beneficial" nutrients or nutrients to limit, or be a combination of these? Or, as we discussed before, should the focus be on food groups instead of nutrients? There are pros and cons to each approach. The pro of all of these indices is that it provides a numeric score connecting food, nutrition, and health, which reduces the informational density and eases decision making. The con is all of the questions above and more generally is its subjective nature (i.e., lack of agreement on which nutrients or foods to emphasize). Furthermore, related to diet, the indices usually do not take into account how often the food is consumed, where, and in what context.

Table 1.5 shows a range of nutrition indices available to evaluate individual foods and diets. As you can see, there are many different aspects to them, depending on what you want to consider or what you value—such as specific nutrients or possible use.

TABLE 1.5

Examples of Numeric Nutrition Indexes

Index	Equation/Calculation	Nutrients of Interest	Application/Use	Nutrient, Food, or Diet	Quality Versus Quantity	Example
Dietary Reference Intakes[a]	Recommended Daily Allowance (RDA): Average daily nutrient intake level that meets the needs of nearly all (97–98%) healthy people in a particular life stage and gender group	Includes levels for all individual macro- and micronutrients	Individual counseling; Development of Dietary Guidelines for Americans, MyPlate, Nutrition Facts Label	Individual nutrients	Quality	RDA Vitamin C: 75 mg/day for females, 19–30 years old
Calories (kcal) (food)[b]	No calculation: simply calories within a food	Calories	Nutrition Facts Label, menu labeling	Individual food	Quantity	1 mango: 100 kcal 1 large chocolate-chip cookie: margarine: 100 kcal
Calories (kcal) (diet)[b]	Sum the calories (kcal) of all foods and beverages within a 24-hour period (or other specified time period).	Calories	Assessment	Diet	Quantity	2,100 kcal/day for moderately active female 19–30 years old
Nutrient density[c]	Divide the amount of a nutrient per 100 g and divide by the RDA for that nutrient, based on age and gender.	Select nutrient	Research	Individual food	Quality	Vitamin C in mango: 0.37 (mango contains 27.7 mg/100 g; RDA based on female, 19–30 years old) Vitamin C in chocolate-chip cookie: 0
Energy density (food)[d]	Ratio of energy (kcal) per weight of food	Calories (kcal)	Research	Individual food	Quantity and quality	Mango: 0.65 kcal/g Chocolate-chip cookie: 6.5 kcal/g

Term	Definition		Application		Quantity and quality	Example
Energy density (diet)[d]	Ratio of energy (kcal or kJ) per weight of all foods consumed in a day. There are various ways to calculate, with no agreed-upon method: food only; all energy-yielding foods and beverages; and all foods and beverages.[j]	Calories (kcal or kilojoules)	Research	Diet		8.03 kJ/g (food only) 3.84 kJ/g (energy-yielding foods and beverages) 5.45 kJ/g (all foods and beverages)[j]
Daily value[e]	Nutrient for individual food (based on serving size)/RDA for Food times 100	Any nutrient of interest	Nutrition Facts Label	Diet	Quality	Mango: 96% of vitamin C (full mango)
Healthy Eating Index[f]	Sum of 10 dietary components with a maximum score of 100 (optimal): total fruit, whole fruit, total vegetables, greens and beans, whole grains, dairy, total protein foods, seafood and plant proteins, fatty acids, refined grains, sodium, empty calories	Food groups, nutrient density	Assessment, research	Diet	Quality	63.8[f] (based on 1994–1996

(continued)

TABLE 1.5
Continued

Index	Equation/Calculation	Nutrients of Interest	Application/Use	Nutrient, Food, or Diet	Quality Versus Quantity	Example
Food Security[g]	Classification based on responses to affirmative questions in Food Security Module. Classifications include high food security, marginal food security, low food security, and very low food security.	Not nutrient-focused, but food sufficiency. Questions pertain to uncertainty about "running out of food," hunger, restricting eating, and eating a "balanced meal."	Assessment, research	Diet	Quantity, a little quality	Food security
NuVal[h]	Unpublished algorithm (patent pending) with scores from 1 with 100 being optimal	Numerous nutrients	Food packaging	Food	Quality	Mango: 100 Chocolate-chip cookie: 1

[a] U.S. Department of Agriculture, National Agricultural Library 2015.
[b] U.S. Department of Agriculture, Agricultural Research Service 2014.
[c] Berner et al. 2001, Darmon et al. 2005.
[d] Vernarelli et al. 2013.
[e] U.S. Food and Drug Administration 2015a.
[f] U.S. Department of Agriculture, Center for Nutrition Policy and Promotion 2015.
[g] U.S. Department of Agriculture, Economic Research Service 2015a.
[h] NuVal 2015.
[i] Energy-yielding beverages include milk, sugar-sweetened beverages, and alcohol.
[j] Averages across a sample of Americans (Frazao 1999).

Summary

Nutrition is a key factor in health promotion and disease prevention. Considering the fact that nutrients can be found across different foods and the number of foods available on the market, understanding how to make choices related to nutrition is extremely complicated. Mathematical equations and indices can be used to compare and contrast nutrients across foods and beverages, meals, and the total diet. However, founded on the DRIs, the Nutrition Facts Label, MyPlate, and the DGAs are designed to simplify nutrition so that people can more easily make decisions to optimize their nutrition.

Closing Conversation

Margaret: Thank you. I learned a lot about nutrition. Economics seems simple and straightforward to me compared to nutrition.

JP: I wish it were simpler. It would make healthy eating simpler too!

Margaret: When I was growing up, I don't remember hearing much about nutrition. Why is that?

JP: Come on. Let's go to the next session where that is to be discussed.

2

Food, Nutrients, and Health
SOME DATA

Learning Objectives

What you will know by the end of this chapter:

◻ key vital statistics used to monitor and describe a population's health status;
◻ national trends in food consumption and dietary intake;
◻ nutrition-related diseases and conditions; and
◻ social determinants of health.

Opening Conversation

JP (at the session): Nutrition is a relatively new field. Each day we learn new things about how nutrients work in our bodies. There is also a lot more information on what people are eating now and how that affects our health.

Margaret: The popular press gives the impression that people are not eating well. Is that true?

JP: It really depends on what food groups and nutrients you look at.

Margaret: How do you know?

JP: I think the speaker will cover that.

Background

Chapter 1 provided an overview of nutrition, including different types of nutrients, the relationship between nutrition and health, different approaches to analyze the nutritional profile of foods and meals, and tools to help simplify food choices and optimize nutrition. What do we know about how Americans are doing in regard to nutrition? And how do we know this?

National Nutrition Data

Let's begin with the "how." Much of what we know about Americans' diets is obtained through a coordinated and comprehensive national monitoring and surveillance program called the U.S. National Nutrition Monitoring and Related Research Program (NNMRRP) (Interagency Board for Nutrition Monitoring and Related Research 2000). The primary goals of the program's monitoring and surveillance systems are to collect continuous, timely, and reliable data to help inform nutrition programs and policies and to track progress toward national nutrition and health objectives. These systems include the National Health and Nutrition Examination Survey (NHANES) and the Behavioral Risk Factor Surveillance System. Ongoing analyses are also conducted to assess nutrients in different and emerging foods and beverages available in the United States. All analyzed items are in the U.S. Department of Agriculture nutrient database (U.S. Department of Agriculture, Agricultural Research Service 2014). Although not officially part of the NNMRRP, the Food Security Module, part of the Current Population Survey directed by the U.S. Census Bureau, is also a key national survey to monitor the prevalence of food insecurity within the United States.

Each of these surveys has different objectives, target populations, and methods for collecting data. Together, they help paint a picture of the American food and dietary behavior landscape. It is important to note that while these surveys are designed to provide an overarching view of diet and health in the United States, data are collected and presented in different ways, so they are not necessarily uniform.

Food Consumption and Dietary Intake

Now for the "what." Although we know what we *should* eat (based on the DRIs, MyPlate, and the DGAs; you may want to refer to Table 1.2), "what" we *do* eat (based on what we know from different monitoring and surveillance tools, as well as research studies) looks much different. Overall, Americans are not meeting most of the goals for key nutrients or recommendations outlined in these food and nutrition–based guides. In general, Americans consume excessive amounts of certain nutrients—such as sodium/salt, (animal) protein, saturated/solid fats, and added sugars—and do not consume enough of other nutrients—such as calcium, vitamin D, fiber, and potassium (U.S. Department of Health and Human Services 2015). Correspondingly, in regard to food groups, the U.S. population has low intakes of fruit, vegetables, whole grains, and dairy. Furthermore, population intake is too high for refined grains, and sodium and saturated fat are overconsumed. Table 2.1 extends Table 1.2 and summarizes general food consumption and dietary intake relative to recommendations by key nutrient and food group. When we examine adherence to all recommendations combined, the results are even more staggering: only between 0% and 33.6% of individuals follow all of the recommendations (Haack and Byker 2014).

TABLE 2.1

Consumption of Key Nutrients Relative to Recommendations

Class of Nutrient	Specific Nutrient	Function	Food Source	Primary Food Group(s) of MyPlate	Consumption[a,b]
					⇑ = Exceeds recommendations
					⇓ = Does not meet recommendations
					⇔ = Meets recommendations (optimal)
Macronutrient	Carbohydrates	Primary energy source for the brain	Complex carbohydrates ◻ Bread ◻ Pasta ◻ Potatoes ◻ Rice ◻ Vegetables Simple sugars ◻ Naturally in fruit ◻ Added to sodas/soft drinks, fruit drinks, desserts, and candy	Grains	⇔ for total grains ⇓ for whole grains
Macronutrient	Fat	Energy source and energy storage Also helps increase the absorption of fat-soluble vitamins and precursors (e.g., vitamin A)	◻ Butter ◻ Margarine ◻ Vegetable oil ◻ Grain-based desserts (cookies, cake, pie) ◻ Pizza ◻ Cheese ◻ Fatty meats like sausages and bacon ◻ French fries	Naturally in protein (fatty sources of animal protein) and dairy (unless nonfat or low-fat), but can be added to foods in all food groups	⇔ for total fat ⇑ for saturated fat ⇔ for trans fat

(continued)

TABLE 2.1
Continued

Class of Nutrient	Specific Nutrient	Function	Food Source	Primary Food Group(s) of MyPlate	Consumption[a,b] ⇑ = Exceeds recommendations ⇓ = Does not meet recommendations ⇔ = Meets recommendations (optimal)
Macronutrient	Protein and amino acids (building blocks of protein)	Provide structure to the body Function as enzymes and sometimes hormones	Animal sources ◻ Beef ◻ Pork ◻ Chicken ◻ Fish ◻ Eggs ◻ Dairy products Vegetable sources ◻ Dried beans/legumes ◻ Grains ◻ Seeds ◻ Nuts	Protein	⇑ for meat sources ⇓ for dried beans/legumes, seeds, and nuts
Vitamin	Vitamin A *Fat-soluble*	Night vision and prevention of disease	◻ Brightly colored fruits ◻ Leafy green vegetables ◻ Meat ◻ Dairy products ◻ Fortified ready-to-eat cereals (read the Nutrition Facts Label)	Fruits and vegetables	⇓

					⇔ for total grains ⇩ for whole grains
Vitamin	Vitamin B-1 (thiamin, aneurin), vitamin B-2 (riboflavin), Vitamin B-3 (niacin), vitamin B-5 (pantothenic acid), Vitamin B-6 (pyridoxal, pyridoxine, pyridoxamine), Vitamin B-12 (cobalamin), folate (folic acid)	Help with energy utilization	¤ Meat ¤ Fish ¤ Dairy products ¤ Dried beans/legumes ¤ Fortified ready-to-eat cereals ¤ Whole-grain products ¤ Bread and bread products	Grains	
Vitamin	Vitamin C (ascorbic acid)	Heals wounds, builds connective tissue, helps with iron absorption	¤ Dairy products ¤ Corn tortillas ¤ Calcium-fortified tofu ¤ Chinese cabbage ¤ Kale ¤ Broccoli ¤ Calcium-fortified foods and beverages (e.g., orange juice, soy milk)	Dairy	⇨
Vitamin	Vitamin D (calciferol) *Fat-soluble*	Assists with calcium absorption and promotes bone health	¤ Fortified dairy ¤ Bread and grain products ¤ Sunshine (when ultraviolet rays from sunlight hit the skin, vitamin D is made)	Dairy	⇨
Vitamin	Vitamin E (α-tocopherol) *Fat-soluble*	Protects tissues from oxidation	¤ Wheat germ ¤ Nuts and seeds ¤ Vegetable oils ¤ Fruit	Grains and protein	⇨

(continued)

TABLE 2.1
Continued

Class of Nutrient	Specific Nutrient	Function	Food Source	Primary Food Group(s) of MyPlate	Consumptiona,b ⇑ = Exceeds recommendations ⇓ = Does not meet recommendations ⇔ = Meets recommendations (optimal)
Vitamin	Vitamin K (derived from German word *koagulation*) *Fat-soluble*	Helps with the function and synthesis of many proteins involved in blood clotting and bone metabolism	¤ Green leafy vegetables (collards, kale, spinach, Swiss chard, salad greens, broccoli) ¤ Dark berries ¤ Vegetable oils and margarine	Vegetables	⇓
Mineral	Calcium	Bone and tooth formation, role in blood clotting and nerve transmission	¤ Dairy products ¤ Corn tortillas ¤ Calcium-fortified tofu ¤ Chinese cabbage ¤ Kale ¤ Broccoli ¤ Calcium-fortified foods and beverages (e.g., orange juice, soy milk)	Dairy	⇓
Mineral	Iron	Helps build red blood cells along with protein to carry oxygen throughout the body	¤ Meat ¤ Fortified bread and grain products ¤ Fruits ¤ Vegetables	Protein	⇑
Mineral	Magnesium	Aids in production of energy; helps muscles, arteries, and heart function properly	¤ Vegetables ¤ Wheat bran ¤ Nuts	Vegetables	⇓

				Food group	
Mineral	Potassium	Helps muscles contract and nerves communicate; aids in regulation of blood pressure	¤ Leafy greens (spinach and collard greens) ¤ Fruit from vines like blackberries and grapes ¤ Root vegetables (carrots, potatoes) ¤ Dairy products	Vegetables	⇨
Mineral	Zinc	Helps the immune system (fighting infection, wound healing), synthesizes proteins and DNA Involved in gene regulation Considered an immune promoter	¤ Red meats ¤ Certain seafood and fish ¤ Fortified ready-to-eat cereals	Fruits, vegetables, and (whole) grains	⇦
Other	Fiber	Aids with digestive health	¤ Whole grains (oats, wheat, unmilled rice, etc.) ¤ Fresh fruits ¤ Fresh vegetables	Fruits, vegetables, and (whole) grains	⇨
Other	Water	Helps transport nutrients and oxygen to cells	All water contained in food, beverages, and drinking water	Water	⇨

[a] These designations are based on overall trends, not necessarily across all age and sociodemographic groups. Designations may be different for different nutrients within the same food group, depending on the food sources. Also, note that "exceeds" is considered a negative behavior, not a positive one.
[b] U.S. Department of Health and Human Services 2010, 2015.

Remember in Chapter 1 when we presented the different indices as ways to "quantify" nutrition? Well, one of the more popular indices from the list is the Healthy Eating Index (HEI) (Ervin 2011). It is an assessment tool designed to look at overall dietary quality, including fruits, vegetables, grains, sodium, and solid fats and added sugars. The maximum possible score is 100; the higher the score, the better a person is doing. Studies using the HEI have found that the average score for children 2 to 17 years old was 49.8, not even half of the total possible score (U.S. Department of Agriculture, Center for Nutrition Policy and Promotion 2013). Dairy and protein were the closest to the standards, and greens, beans, and whole grains were the farthest. Based on an older version of the HEI, adults scored below the maximum score for all components except total grains and meats and beans (Ervin 2011). Similar to children, the scores for dark green and orange vegetables and legumes, whole grains, sodium, and calories from solid fats and added sugars were low, less than half of the possible score.

It is important to note that these results are presented as population-based averages, meaning they are to represent the whole country. What does that mean? That means that some individuals may do a whole lot better and follow many and/or all of the recommendations—but others may do even worse. There are differences based on:

Age (children eat more fruit, drink more milk, consume more added sugars, and eat fewer vegetables and whole grains than adults),

Gender (adult women usually eat more whole grains, fruits, and vegetables, and less saturated fat than men),

Race/ethnicity (non-Hispanic white and Mexican-American individuals report higher dietary quality than non-Hispanic black persons),

Income and education (individuals with higher income and/or educational levels, such as more than a high school education, generally eat better),

Geography (residents of the southern states tend to have lower adherence to dietary recommendations than those in other regions, like the western states), and

Community (some communities do not have healthy foods available, such as many lower-income neighborhoods and rural areas).

(Johnston, Poti, and Popkin 2014; Leung et al. 2014; U.S. Department of Health and Human Services 2015; Wang et al. 2014).

These trends also translate to overall health outcomes and behaviors. For example, whites individuals have more favorable health profiles than individuals of other races and ethnicities, except for Asian individuals, who have similar or better health profiles (Nguyen, Moser, and Chou 2014). What are some reasons you think may account for these differences? What underlying factors appear consistent across these categories? (Hint: economics.)

Nutrition-Related Chronic Conditions and Diseases

If individuals are not meeting nutrient, food, or nutrition recommendations, in terms of both under-consumption and overconsumption, what does that mean for Americans' health status? As we introduced in Chapter 1, about half of all American adults have one or more preventable chronic diseases. Based on data from the NNMRRP, which also collects information on key vital statistics, we know that the prevalence and incidence of many nutrition-related conditions and diseases in the United States have increased over the past 20 years. *Prevalence* is the percentage of a population that is affected by a particular condition or disease at a given time. *Incidence* is the rate of occurrence of a particular condition or disease. Furthermore, scientific evidence (you may want to review Table 1.4 again) has shown that poor dietary patterns directly contribute to health, weight status, and chronic disease (Table 2.2).

What are some things you notice? Which foods or nutrients consistently lower the risk of conditions or diseases? If you said fruits and vegetables, you are correct. Think now about MyPlate and what portion should consist of fruits and vegetables. This should help you connect the foods with the reason—health. Which foods or nutrients increase the risk? If you think solid fats and added sugars, again you are correct. And this is precisely why you don't see them at all in MyPlate and why these nutrients are featured in the Nutrition Facts Label—so consumers can try to limit them. Alcohol should also be limited as it provides little in the way of nutritional value. Finally, how serious are these diseases? It's time to provide a brief overview of the leading nutrition-related conditions and diseases.

OVERWEIGHT AND OBESITY

Recent data show that 31.8% of children (2–19 years old) are either overweight or obese and 16.9% are obese (Ogden et al. 2014). More than two-thirds (68.5%) of adults are considered overweight or obese, 34.9% obese, and 6.4% extremely obese, based on 2011–2012 NHANES data. Overweight and obesity refer to body weights that exceed what is considered healthy or optimal for an individual. Currently, overweight and obesity are determined by body mass index (BMI), intended to correlate to body fatness. High levels of body fatness have been strongly associated with type 2 diabetes, high blood pressure, atherosclerosis, heart disease, stroke, and certain types of cancer. BMI is computed by dividing weight in pounds (lb) by height in inches (in) squared and multiplying by a conversion factor of 703: weight (lb)/[height (in)]^2 × 703. BMI is used differently for children than for adults (Table 2.3). For children and adolescents, BMI-for-age is plotted on gender-specific growth charts developed by the Centers for Disease Control and Prevention (Centers for Disease and Prevention. Division of Nutrition, Physical Activity, and Obesity 2015). These charts track a child's BMI in relation to those of other children of the same gender and age. For adults, overweight or obesity is determined by cutoffs.

TABLE 2.2

Dietary Risk Factors Associated with the Prevention of the Leading Causes of Death[a]

Food and Beverage Categories	Specific	Leading Causes and Contributors of Death							
		Obesity	Heart Disease	Stroke	Diabetes (Type 2)[b]	Cancer	High Blood Pressure	Osteoporosis[c]	Accidents, Unintentional Injuries
Grains	Whole grains		↓	↓	↓	↓	↓		
Vegetables		↓	↓	↓	↓	↓	↓		
Fruit		↓	↓	↓	↓	↓	↓		
Dairy	Low-fat dairy	↓	↓					↓	
Protein	Processed and/or fatty meats	↑	↑			↑			
Added Sugars	Sugar-sweetened beverages, grain-based desserts	↑	↑ triglycerides		↑				
Fats and Oils	Saturated/solid fats and trans fasts	↑	↑	↑	↑	↑	↑		
Alcohol	Excessive intake	↑	↑	↑		↑	↑		↑

[a] Based on the USDA Nutrition Evidence Library 2014 "moderate" or "significant" associations.

[b] Comorbid factor for high blood pressure, high cholesterol, heart disease and stroke; obesity a risk factor. Type 1 diabetes cannot be prevented and is therefore not listed here.

[c] Through unintentional injuries in aging audiences.

TABLE 2.3

Weight Classifications and BMI for Children and Adults[a]

Weight Classification	Child	Adult
Underweight	BMI for age and gender <5th percentile	<18.5
Healthy	BMI for age and gender 5th to 85th percentile	18.5–24.9
Overweight	BMI for age and gender 85th percentile to <95th percentile	25.0–29.9
Obese	BMI for age and gender ≥95th percentile	≥30

[a] Centers for Disease Control and Prevention. Division of Nutrition, Physical Activity, and Obesity 2015.

Maintaining a healthy weight is about balancing what and how much a person eats and drinks (calories in) with how much energy the person uses in day-to-day activities and physical movement (calories out). Consuming a diet consistent with MyPlate that is rich in whole grains, fruits, vegetables, low-fat dairy, and lean meats or beans will help achieve a healthy weight, along with limiting solid fats and added sugars, such as sugar-sweetened beverages.

HEART DISEASE

Heart disease is the leading cause of death in the United States. Deaths attributed to heart disease account for one of every four deaths (Centers for Disease Control and Prevention, National Center for Health Statistics 2014). There are several different types of heart disease, including coronary artery disease and stroke. Coronary heart disease is the most common type of heart disease. It has been estimated that at least 200,000 deaths from heart disease and stroke each year could be prevented (Centers for Disease Control and Prevention 2013). The development and progression of heart disease are attributed to atherosclerosis, the hardening of arteries, "tubes" within the circulatory system that transport blood (with oxygen) from the heart to the entire body. Atherosclerosis usually begins with the accumulation of soft, fatty streaks along the inner walls of the arteries called *plaque*.

It is not known exactly how it begins or even the exact causes, but it is known that certain behaviors increase the likelihood, such as solid fats. Think about pouring melted butter down your kitchen drain. What happens? It sticks to the side of the pipes. If you wait long enough, (hot) water may help wash it down some. But if you did this a few times a day and every day, you would need to call a plumber. What else could you do? You could add lemon juice and break down some of the fat. Now replace pipes with arteries; butter with butter, creamy soft cheese, ice cream, bacon and other processed meats, and anything else high in solid fats; plumber with cardiologist; and lemon juice with fruits, vegetables, whole grains, and nuts. The fiber in the fruits, vegetables, whole grains, and nuts, as well as many vitamins and minerals that are considered *antioxidants*, help bind to cholesterol and get it out of your body before it can do damage. Nuts also contain beneficial or "good" fats that do not contribute to clogging of the arteries.

DIABETES

In 2012, 29.1 million Americans, or 9.3% of the population, had diabetes (American Diabetes Association 2014). Since 1990, the prevalence of diagnosed diabetes in the United States rose sharply (Centers for Disease Control and Prevention 2012). It increased by at least 50% in 42 states and by at least 100% in 18 states. The prevalence and incidence of diabetes are increasing, in part due to increasing rates of overweight and obesity. There are two types of diabetes: type 1 and type 2. Type 1 is when the beta cells within the pancreas no longer make *insulin*. Insulin is a hormone that helps the body use glucose and starches, including grains, for energy. Individuals with type 1 diabetes need to inject insulin. Type 2 is when the body does not make enough insulin or cannot use insulin properly, resulting in limited utilization of blood glucose. Type 1 often occurs in childhood and cannot be prevented. Type 2 diabetes, on the other hand, occurs more frequently in adulthood and can be prevented. Overweight and obesity, including poor diet and physical inactivity, are the leading risk factors for type 2 diabetes.

CANCER

Cancer is a term to describe a group of diseases that cause the uncontrolled growth and spread of abnormal cells. Cancer cells can spread to other parts of the body through the circulatory system. Cancer is not just one disease: there are actually more than 100 different types of cancer. Cancer is the second leading cause of death for Americans. In 2014, 585,720 Americans are expected to die from it (1,600 people per day), and another 1,665,540 new cancer cases will be diagnosed (American Cancer Society 2014). Prostate and breast cancer will be diagnosed at the highest rate for men and women, respectively, but lung and bronchus cancer is the top contributor to cancer deaths for both men and women, based on estimates.

There are a wide variety of risk factors for each type or location of cancer, but research shows that the following risk factors are consistent across cancer types: tobacco use, excessive alcohol intake, excessive exposure to ultraviolet rays (for skin cancer), and an unhealthy diet. In fact, it has been estimated that one-quarter to one-third of cancers in countries such as the United States are due to poor nutrition, physical inactivity, and overweight/obesity (American Cancer Society 2014; World Cancer Research Fund 2007). Diet recommendations for cancer prevention emphasize the consumption of plant foods, including a diet rich in fruits and vegetables and whole grains, and limiting the consumption of red and processed meat. Alcohol consumption should also be limited to one drink per day for women and two for men.

HIGH BLOOD PRESSURE

Nearly 67 million Americans (31%) have high blood pressure, one of every three adults, and another one in three have prehypertension (Nwankwo et al. 2013). High blood pressure is considered one of the risk factors for heart disease and stroke. Blood pressure is the pressure of the blood in the circulatory system. Blood pressure provides diagnostic information on the "health" of the heart and arteries. Elevated or high blood pressure (stage 1) is also known as hypertension and refers to a blood pressure measurement of more than 140 mm Hg systolic or more than 90 mm Hg diastolic. There are several risk factors for hypertension that are similar to those for heart disease: overweight/obesity, stress, use of tobacco, excessive alcohol intake, excessive sodium intake, and inadequate potassium intake.

To address possible effects of hypertension, the Dietary Approaches to Stop Hypertension (DASH) diet has been recommended, based on numerous studies (Epstein et al. 2012). The diet emphasizes fruit, vegetables, whole grains, fat-free or low-fat dairy products, beans, nuts, and fish and poultry. Nuts, fish, and poultry have healthy, not saturated/solid, fats. Individuals should also limit sodium/salt, sweets, sugary beverages, and red meats like beef.

OSTEOPOROSIS

Osteoporosis is a disease in which the bones are weak and not as healthy as desired.. They instead are considered "porous" (*osteo* = bone; *poros* = porous) and weak and may break as a result of falls or injuries. It takes place when a person doesn't make enough bone mass (until adulthood) or loses too much (during the aging process). Although it is not as much of a public health focus as the other diseases and conditions, about 54 million Americans have osteoporosis and low bone mass, meaning they are at increased risk for osteoporosis (National Osteoporosis Foundation 2014). Breaking a bone can seriously impair a person's quality of life and is extremely serious for seniors in particular. Recommendations for ensuring bone health include consuming enough calcium and vitamin D (dairy) and eating a well-balanced diet, as shown by MyPlate. Regular physical activity is also important, including weight-bearing exercise. Smoking should be avoided and alcohol limited as well.

FOOD SECURITY

Although it's not a health condition or a disease, *food security*—access by all people at all times to enough food for an active, healthy life—is an important "condition" for a healthy population free of disease. It can also be considered a different type of index or measure and was included in Table 1.5. Most households (85.7%) in the United States have consistent and reliable access to enough food (Coleman-Jensen, Gregory, and Singh 2014), but 14.3%, or 17.5 million households, do not. They are considered food insecure—either low or very low food. Historically, most emergency food and nutrition assistance programs have focused on increasing the amount of food (i.e., calories), not necessarily the quality of food (i.e., calories and nutrients). The biggest predictor of food insecurity is household income: individuals living in poverty are at higher risk for food insecurity (Gundersen, Kreider, and Pepper 2011). Later in the book, we will review some scenarios that may influence food choices among low-income and food-insecure audiences.

With the other health conditions and diseases, there were dietary trends that contributed to the condition or state. For food security, there are not dietary trends that contribute per se to food security. There are dietary trends that are consequences of food insecurity, however. Individuals who suffer from hunger and food insecurity tend to have diets higher in total fat, solid fats, added sugars, and sodium and lower in whole grains, fruits, and vegetables, which may ultimately lead to chronic diseases and conditions (Leung et al. 2014). Why do you think this may be the case?

HEALTH DISPARITIES

Many of the health concerns and diseases we just reviewed affect certain populations at higher proportions. These disproportions are often referred to as *health disparities*. Race or ethnicity, sex, sexual identity, age, disability, education, income, and geographic location all contribute to an individual's ability to achieve good health (Healthy People 2020 2015). Controlling for these differences, the largest cluster of risk factors for these conditions and disease is overall dietary quality, similar to the trends we reported earlier.

Summary

Currently, there are many shortfalls between the food and nutrition–based guidelines discussed in Chapter 1 and the dietary intake patterns and trends among Americans that help portray the health of our nation. Significant improvements are required to optimize health and prevent many of the conditions and diseases we discussed, such as overweight and obesity, type 2 diabetes, and heart disease. Throughout the remainder of the book, we will provide insights into a number of economic factors that may help explain these patterns and also help guide initiatives, interventions, and even policies to encourage healthy eating.

Closing Conversation

Margaret: I see now how important food and nutrition are for our public's health. There is a lot of overlap too for risk factors for the different diseases and conditions.

JP: Yes, there definitely is. There is also overlap in who is at risk for these diseases and conditions.

Margaret: I see now how we could be good partners. Economics plays a role in what people eat.

JP: Can you tell me more—but first, can we eat?

Margaret: Sure, now I know what I "should" eat. I can tell you a little more about economics during dinner.

PART II

The Economics of Food Consumption

This section of the book covers the economics of food consumption. Chapters 3 through 7 provide a neoclassical treatment of the economics of food consumption. The neoclassical economics of food consumption rest on four building blocks, which are introduced in Chapter 3 in the context of the effect of income when there is only one food and one nutrient. This simplification helps solidify the understanding of the building blocks. Chapter 4 extends the analysis in Chapter 3 to allow for substitution between foods while again focusing on the effect of income. The framework is used to derive the Engle curve, which shows the relationship between income and food consumption. Chapter 5 uses the Chapter 4 framework but shifts the focus to analyzing how prices affect food and nutrition choices. This leads to a derivation and discussion of the law of demand. Chapter 6 adds a convenience and time dimension to the analysis of Chapter 5, taking into account not only the money price of a food item but also its time price. The chapter discusses how convenience and time constraints affect the demand for food. Chapter 7 incorporates the role of information, such as advertising or a nutrition education program, into the economic framework developed in Chapters 3 through 6. This chapter shows how information may affect preferences and therefore influence the demand for foods. Chapter 8 provides the economic framework for analyzing the tradeoffs between rewards received from eating a food now (what are called hedonic effects) versus the possible later health rewards or cost. The analysis shows why there is a tendency to place little value on future health rewards and therefore a tendency to eat too much unhealthy savory food now. Chapter 9 gives an overview of behavioral economics and discusses eight major behavioral economic effects that would seem especially relevant for food and nutrition choices. Chapter 10 places both the neoclassical and behavioral economic approaches under the broader unifying framework of neuroeconomics. This broader framework sheds new light on why some factors may seem more important than others and why some interventions may be more effective than others. Chapters 3 through 10 contain some of the main empirical findings in the context of food related to the economic factor discussed in the chapter.

3

Income and the Foundations

Learning Objectives

What you will know by the end of this chapter:

¤ the foundations of consumer choice within a food and nutrition context; and

¤ how food, nutrients, budget, and preferences interact to determine food and nutrient choices in relation to recommendations.

Opening Conversation

Margaret: Before we get started, is JP short for anything?

JP: It is. I'm named after both of my parents' fathers—Jon Paul.

Margaret: I was interested to hear about changes in dietary behavior and health by different groups of individuals, especially individuals with different incomes. The relationship between income and choices is one of the main areas of interest to economists.

JP: I thought you may be interested in that. Yes, income appears to drive many different food decisions, but it seems complicated to me. Does economics provide a systematic framework for analysis?

Margaret: Yes, it does. It is a rather intricate framework, so I think it will help to start with a very simple, and yes unrealistic, case of one food and one nutrient.

Some Data on Food Expenditures and Income

Even casual observations suggest that food and nutrition choices are affected by money. For this book, the amount of money a person, family, and/or household has to spend will be called *income or budget*. What is the empirical relationship between spending on food and income? Figure 3.1 shows food consumption expenditures on four general food groups by income quintiles in the United States for 2012. Quintiles come from sorting and separating the data by income into five

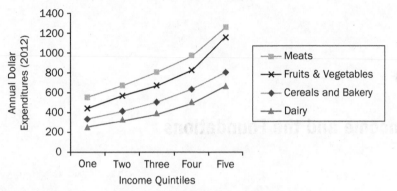

FIGURE 3.1. Major Food Group Expenditures by Income Quintiles (2012).
Source: Bureau of Labor Statistics, Consumer Expenditure Survey 2012.

equal parts: the lowest (first) 20%, the next lowest (second) 20%, the third 20%, the fourth 20%, and the fifth 20% (highest). The quintiles correspond to average annual household after-tax incomes of \$10,171, \$27,743, \$46,777, \$73,970, and \$158,024, respectively. Figure 3.1 reveals that as income goes up, food purchases also go up—a positive relationship. Across all income groups more money is spent on meat, then fruits and vegetables, then cereals and bakery, and finally dairy. These are the categories used by the Bureau of Labor Statistics and are different from those used by MyPlate. As Kirkpatrick et al. (2012) show, actual food intake and adherence to dietary guidelines also improve with income.

The Economic Foundations of Food Choices with One Food and One Nutrient

While basic intuition suggests that nutrition and health improve with income, we can all think of counter-examples where someone with a high income does not eat in a very healthy way. Consequently, the interaction among income, food, and health is more intricate than basic intuition would suggest. The economic approach bases this interaction on four building blocks:

1. The food–nutrient relationship,
2. The food–budget relationship,
3. The nutrient–health relationship, and
4. The food–preference relationship.

Once these four building blocks are put together, we have a unified foundational framework that can be used to explore numerous food and nutrition choice scenarios.

   To keep the focus on the economic concepts, we start with the overly simplistic case of one food and one nutrient—what we will refer to as a 1 food × 1 nutrient model. The objective here is to learn the fundamentals. Think of the 1 × 1 model as an appetizer consisting of all the ingredients and techniques you will need in preparing more complicated recipes. Chapter 4 will extend the analysis to more than one food.

Before we get started, all concepts in this chapter will be presented using all four languages: numeric, graphical, mathematical, and verbal. These are all complementary languages, but the most powerful at this foundational level is the graphical. You should strive to become fluent in the graphical language—that is, being able to read and manipulate the graphs.

The Food–Nutrient Relationship

As discussed in Chapter 1, if we know the amount of a food consumed in grams we can calculate the number of grams of a nutrient. Figure 3.2 shows the food–nutrient

Ground Beef (g)	Protein (g)
0	0
100	24
200	48
250	60
300	72

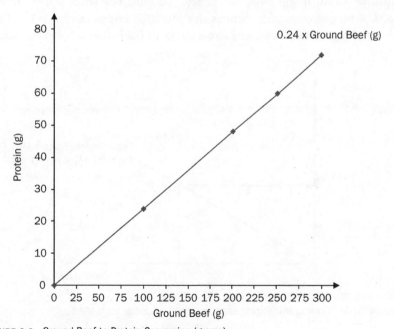

FIGURE 3.2. Ground Beef-to-Protein Conversion (grams).

relationship for ground beef (regular, broiled) to protein. The *recommended* intake of protein per day for males 19 to 30 years old is 56 grams (see Table 1.2). If we round up to 60 grams and acquire all protein from ground beef, this corresponds to about 250 grams (see the highlighted row). The line connecting the data points quickly conveys the positive relationship between grams of hamburger and grams of protein. The slope of the line is the protein conversion factor for a gram of ground beef (0.24).

Let's now generalize Figure 3.2. With one food and one nutrient, the nutrient conversion formula from Chapter 1 is simply

$$N_1 = \alpha_{11}F_1 : Food - Nutrient\ Relationship \tag{3.1}$$

F_1 would be grams of ground beef (100, 200, 250, 300), $\alpha_{11} = 0.24$, and N_1 would be the amount of protein (24, 48, 60, 72).

The transition graph (numbers and symbols) in Figure 3.3 shows the general representation of Equation 3.1. Note because of the one-to-one relationship between the food (F_1) and the nutrient (N_1), the recommended levels of the nutrient and food are then represented by N_1^R and F_1^R, respectively. The "In A Phrase Summary" (IAPS) box summarizes the main point in words what the graph says in an Figure 3.3.

The Food–Budget Relationship

If you have more money, you can buy more and/or higher-quality and more expensive goods. If you have less money, you must buy fewer and/or inferior goods. A budget constraint captures this idea. The *budget constraint* is a fixed amount of money to be allocated across all goods (including savings) consumed.

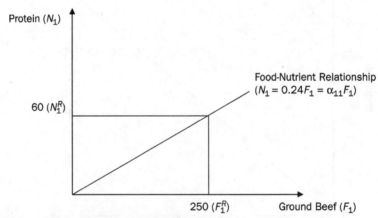

FIGURE 3.3. Recommended Nutrient and Food Levels.
[The IAPS] As food quantity increases, nutrient quantity increases.

Including money you may borrow, you cannot spend more money than you have. The term *goods* includes any items, products, or services that an individual uses or consumes.

Continuing with the regular ground beef example, suppose your budget for ground beef for a day is between $2 and $3. How much ground beef can you buy? According to the Bureau of Labor Statistics in June 2014, the U.S. city average price for ground beef was about $4.00 per pound, which is about $0.01 per gram. So with $2.00 you could buy 200 grams of ground beef ($2.00/0.01), and with $3.00 you could buy 300 grams of ground beef ($3.00/0.01). To reach the recommended level of 250 grams, you will have to spend $2.50.

Consider now the more general relationship. In the case of one food, the budget constraint is written as

$$M = P_1 F_1 : \textit{Food-Budget Relationship,} \tag{3.2}$$

where M is the money level, P_1 is the price of the food item, and F_1 is again the quantity of the food item. Solving for F_1 determines how much you can afford, or

$$F_1 = \frac{M}{P_1} : \textit{Maximum Quantity of Food that can be Purchased} \tag{3.3}$$

Note for any value of F_1 we can substitute Equation 3.3. So we can incorporate the budget constraint into Figure 3.3 using Equation 3.3 to get Figure 3.4. With the low budget of $2.00 ($M^L$ = $2.00, P_1 = 0.01), you can only afford 200 grams of ground beef, which is 48 grams of protein and below the recommended level of 60 grams. The budget is binding with respect to the recommendation level. With the high budget of $3.00 ($M^H$ = $3.00, P_1 = 0.01), you can afford 300 grams of ground

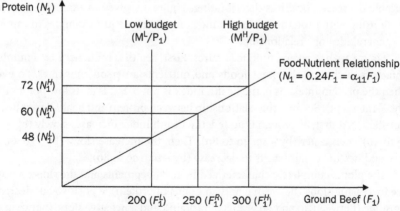

FIGURE 3.4. Recommended Nutrient and Food Levels Associated with Income.
[The IAPS] Budget can determine proximity to recommended levels (N_1^R, F_1^R).

beef, which is 72 grams of protein and above the recommended level. The budget is not binding with respect to the recommendation level.

Let's see how comfortable you are with what we have covered so far.

Some Foundation Building Exercises

1. Suppose there is a *lean* ground beef with a higher protein content per gram than 0.24. How would the food–nutrient relationship in Figure 3.4 change?
2. Given 1, show and explain how you could consume less lean ground beef and still meet the recommended nutrient level.
3. Suppose there is a decrease in the price of *normal* ground beef. What would happen to Figure 3.4?
4. Put your answers to 1 and 3 together on the same graph. Show and explain two alternative ways to hit the nutrient recommendation target: switching to a leaner ground beef given the same budget or paying less for normal ground beef with the existing budget.

The Nutrient–Health Relationship

Let's add the health block. The fundamental premise of nutrition sciences is that good nutrition helps produce good health. In economic terminology, nutrition is an input in the production of health outcomes. The *health production function* shows the technical relationship between inputs and health outcomes. Of course, there are many inputs that affect health, including genetics and lifestyle behaviors like smoking, exercise, and medications, but the focus here is on nutrition. On the output side, there are numerous indicators of health, such as blood pressure or weight status. We will not state specifically how we are measuring health but just label it "health." As the health variable increases, health is improving; as the health variable decreases, health is deteriorating. Figure 3.5 gives an example of such a relationship with protein. The health index numbers are just examples to capture the general idea of a relationship.

Figure 3.5 has several unique features. First, health is influenced by a number of factors, including the other foods and nutrients a person consumes. So even when the protein intake is 0, the health index is not 0, but is at its low point of 30 (the Y intercept). Second, the relationship between protein and health is not linear (constant). At first, as protein is added, the health index increases slowly (by +10, 30 to 40), then faster (by +40, 40 to 80). Then, the increase slows (by +20, 80 to 100) and health actually starts to decrease (by −20, 100 to 80).

The plot is completely characterized by three segments and the slope: a positive increasing slope (between 0 and 40 grams of protein), a positive but decreasing slope (between 40 and 60 grams of protein), and a negative slope (between 60 and 80 grams of protein). A common source of confusion is between a positive but decreasing slope and a negative slope (i.e., decreasing health). They are not the

Health Index	Protein (g)
30	0
40	20
80	40
100	60
80	80

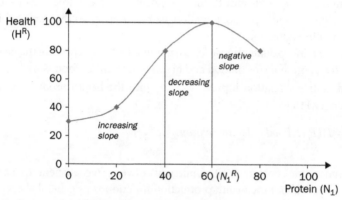

FIGURE 3.5. Unconstrained Health Production Function for Protein.

same. A positive but decreasing slope means the *improvement* in health is getting smaller. A negative slope means health is deteriorating.

Here is an analogy. Think of approaching a stop sign. As you approach a stop sign your change of speed (i.e., the slope) is decreasing, but you are still going forward; you are not going backward. In the nutrient context, at higher amounts, an additional amount of the nutrient does not add as much value to health as at lower amounts. *The health production function will reach its maximum (e.g., 100) where the nutrient is at its recommended level (e.g., 60) or the RDA.* And eventually, beyond a certain point, health may begin to deteriorate. The slope is usually called the *marginal product*.

Nutrient recommendations are also age- and gender-specific, so *different individuals have different health production functions.* This should be intuitive. The same diet can affect different individuals differently. Finally, the health production function in Figure 3.5 is quite general, and *different nutrients or foods will have larger or smaller segments of the curve.* For example, for some nutrients the positive slope region may cover a small range, with a larger range for negative slope (e.g., saturated fat.).

How do we incorporate food and the budget constraint into this analysis? Let's take each in turn. All we need to know about the health production function is that as nutrition improves, health improves in a nonlinear way. Let's express this relationship more compactly so it can be manipulated as

$$H = H(N_1): \textit{Nutrient - Health Relationship} \qquad (3.4)$$
$$\scriptstyle(\pm)$$

Don't be intimidated. This is just a concise little paragraph that says the following. Overall health (H) "is a function of" (that is what the capital H before the paren-thesis means) Nutrient 1, N_1. Over some initial range, as the intake of N_1 increases, health H increases—the little positive sign (+) under N_1. However, at some point as the intake of N_1 continues to increase, health H starts to *decrease*—the little negative sign (–) under N_1. So, Equation 3.4 concisely gives the same information as the graph in Figure 3.5.

However, individuals choose foods, not nutrients, so let's write the health pro-duction function in terms of food and graph it in terms of food. Simply substitute the food–nutrient relationship $N_1 = \alpha_{11}F_1$ into the health production function (Equation 3.4) to yield

$$H = H(F_1): \textit{Food - Health Relationship} \qquad (3.5)$$
$$\scriptstyle(\pm)$$

We can ignore the constant positive nutrient conversion coefficient α_{11}, because all we really know about the health production function is its general shape. A posi-tive constant will not change the general shape.

The budget is incorporated as before by using the relationship $F_1 = M/P_1$. Figure 3.6 shows the budget-constrained health production function. Note that the *unconstrained* maximum health level $H^R(100)$ occurs at the recommended food intake $F_1^R(250)$. Any other level of food intake does not lead to maximum or optimal health. At the low budget ($M^L = \$2.00$, $P_1 = 0.01$), you can afford only 200 grams of ground beef, which leads to a health index of H^L. The budget is a barrier to reaching optimal health H^R. At the high budget ($M^H = \$3.00$, $P_1 = 0.01$),

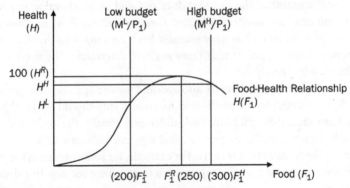

FIGURE 3.6. Budget Constraint and Health Production Function.
[The IAPS] Low budget can prevent reaching recommended food intake and optimal health. A high budget can lead to exceeding the recommendation and result in lower health.

you can afford 300 grams of ground beef, which is greater than the recommended amount and leads to a health index of H^H, which is also *below* the optimal level H^R. What is going on? Too much of a nutrient is not beneficial either, and why we have Upper Intake Levels. In this case, if you are spending your entire budget, then you are consuming beyond the recommended amount, and your health suffers.

The Food-Preference Relationship

If you are perceptive, you have noticed that something very fundamental is missing. Yep, choices. There are no choices. The choice rule is simply that the individual spends all of his or her money on the food item. We need a more general and realistic approach.

Individuals make hundreds of choices every day: what time to get up, what to have for breakfast, where to go to college, whom to date. What is the common objective across all of these activities? You make a decision to try to bring yourself the most satisfaction, given the constraints or barriers you face.

Economists call the metric of your overall satisfaction your *utility*. The idea of utility has a very long history in economics and is based on some rather intuitive insights from human nature. Consider what happens when you are a normal person and start eating a food item you like, such as a hamburger. The first bite tastes really, really good and provides a great deal of satisfaction. The second bite probably also tastes really good and provides satisfaction. The third bite is probably good, but probably not as good as the second one, and the fourth is probably not as good the third, and so forth. The *additional* satisfaction from your final bite of a hamburger will be significantly lower than the first bite. You get "utils" from making choices, but they vary over the choice domain. Note the intuition here is very similar to that of the health production function. You make a choice and consume something (an input), and it produces an output called utility. Consequently, we can proceed in a similar fashion to the health production function.

A *utility function* is a mathematical representation of preferences that shows the relationship between the consumption of goods and the satisfaction received from those goods. The slope of the utility function is called the *marginal utility*, the *addition* to utility of each incremental bite in this case. As long as the marginal utility (slope) is positive, keep consuming more of the good and you will be assured that utility will be increasing. *Diminishing marginal* utility refers to the process of each *additional* unit of consumption providing less *additional* utility than the previous unit. Isn't diminishing marginal utility a universal property of most goods consumed in one sitting, even ice cream or chocolate? Once the marginal utility hits zero, stop consuming (i.e., the last bite of ice cream before you stop).

Just as with the production function, there are a few important facts to keep in mind about the utility function:

- ◻ A utility function represents an individual's preferences or desires.
- ◻ Different individuals have different preferences and therefore different utility functions.
- ◻ There is no common or standard unit for measuring utility. The actual units of utility are not important. What is important is the relative ranking or the ordinality.
- ◻ Utility functions are usually nonlinear.

The most general mathematical form of the utility function is $U = U(q_1, q_2, ..., q_m)$, where U denotes the utility level and the qs are quantities of goods and/or services consumed. However, at this point we are considering just one good, a food, so we will write it initially as

$$U = U(F_1): \textit{Food - Preference Relationship (utility function)} \qquad (3.6)$$
$$\underset{(\pm)}{}$$

Equation 3.6 is read in a similar way to Equation 3.5 for health production. Utility is a function of the amount of food intake. The little + and – signs mean the same as before. Over some range utility is increasing as the food intake F_1 increases. Beyond that range, as the food intake F_1 increases, the utility level U decreases. Maximizing utility subject to a budget constraint looks identical to that of health production and is shown in Figure 3.7. The *unconstrained* maximum utility level $U^u(100)$ occurs at $F_1^u(290 \text{ grams})$. Any other level of food intake does not lead to maximum utility. At the low budget (M^L = $2.00, P_1 = 0.01), you can afford only 200 grams of ground beef, which leads to a utility level of U^L. The budget is a barrier or binding. At the high budget (M^H = $3.00, P_1 = 0.01), you can afford 300 grams of ground beef and get the utility level U^H, which is also *below* the optimal level U^u.

It is important to note that the level of hamburger consumption that maximizes utility $F_1^u(290)$ in Figure 3.7 is *not* the same as the level of hamburger consumption that maximizes health $F_1^R(250)$ in Figure 3.6. This should agree with

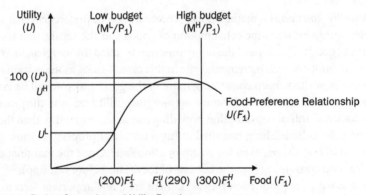

FIGURE 3.7. Budget Constraint and Utility Function.
[The IAPS] A low budget can prevent reaching the maximum utility level.

your intuition. You may enjoy eating a big meat lover's pizza every day, but that is not best for your health. The point? *The optimal food intake for your health is not necessarily the level that gives you the most satisfaction.*

Synapse Stimulants

1. Using Figure 3.6, show what happens to the gap between the recommended food consumption for optimizing *health* and the money-constrained food consumption as price decreases.
2. Using Figure 3.7, show what happens to the gap between the recommended food consumption for optimizing *utility* and the money-constrained food consumption as price decreases.
3. At what point in either Figure 3.6 or 3.7 does the budget or price become irrelevant?

Putting It All Together with Nutrient Recommendation Implications

So how does the consumer choose between optimal health and optimal utility (i.e., satisfaction)? Perhaps you are wondering: yeah, people get satisfaction (utility) from food, but don't they also get utility from health? Where is health in the utility function? Good observation, and indeed we have to incorporate health in the utility function.

Economists, and other disciplines, have long recognized that the goods and services we buy on the market may not directly provide satisfaction but rather are inputs into satisfying more basic wants. For example, when you buy clothes, you may buy them for several reasons, such as staying warm and looking stylish. Food is similar. Food can be consumed for many reasons as well: to counter some emotional experience (e.g., depression), to enhance some social occasion (e.g., a Super Bowl party), and of course to improve health. To keep the analysis manageable, we will follow the literature and consider two aggregate channels: health utility and hedonic utility. *Health utility* refers to all utility from a food that operates through a concern for and evaluation of health effects. *Hedonic utility* will be *any* other source of utility that is not health-related, so would include all sensory components (e.g., smell, texture, taste), emotional, social, and so forth.[1] So the intuition here is that when we eat something, we get utility from the sheer hedonic pleasure of eating the food (e.g., social, smell, taste) and utility from the health benefits (e.g., lower cholesterol, longer life expectancy).

---

[1] Analyzing choices in terms of basic human desires dates back at least to Jeremy Bentham, who was a forefather of utility theory. Bentham claimed there are only about 15 basic "pains" and "pleasures" that determine happiness (Bentham 1963). The formulation here is a simple version of household production theory, made famous by Nobel Laureate Gary Becker and originally applied in the health context by Michael Grossman (Grossman 1972). It is common in the literature to decompose utility arising from two sources: hedonic and utilitarian (e.g., Batra and Ahtola 1991). Given the focus of the book, we use the term *health utility* rather than the broader *utilitarian* term. Furthermore, there is no assumption being made about the hierarchy of preferences between hedonic utility and health. Indeed, economists tend to represent preferences in a very general and global form and are rather agnostic regarding any hierarchy of needs, such as Maslow's hierarchy. Maslow's hierarchy of needs can be shown to be a special case of household production theory presented here (Seeley 1992).

Let's formalize this decomposition of utility into a hedonic and a health component. The hedonic and health effects could interact in numerous ways, but to emphasize the concepts, let us assume they interact in an *additive* fashion such that the utility function (Equation 3.6) is written as

$$U(F_1) = \underset{(\pm)}{h(F_1)} + \underset{(\pm)}{\beta H(F_1)}: \; Total \; Utility \; From \; Food \tag{3.7}$$

The first part, $h(F_1)$, captures the *hedonic* component of utility and the second part, $\beta H(F_1)$, captures the health component of utility. The sum of these is the *total utility function*, which captures all of the components in one equation. The Greek beta (β) simply converts the health units to utility units, and you can think of the β as how much weight the individual places on health in his or her overall utility. This interpretation turns out to be quite useful in later chapters.

Figure 3.8 shows an example of what the total utility function and its components may look like for a specific food and a specific person (age, gender).[2] This figure is an extremely powerful tool for discussing the interaction of food, health, income, prices, and preferences all within a unified framework. True, Figure 3.8 does look rather complicated, but if you review one curve (component) at a time you will see that it is actually very intuitive.

Focus first on the health utility function, $\beta H(F_1)$. As consumption of the food increases, health utility is increasing and reaches a maximum at the recommended level for this food, F_1^R. After F_1^R, the health utility begins to decline. Now look at the hedonic utility function, $h(F_1)$. Note that it continues to increase even after the recommended level F_1^R and does not reach its maximum until F_1^h. If health was no consideration, this person would consume F_1^h. However, health *is* a consideration

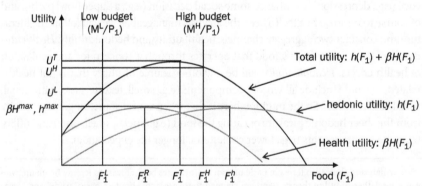

FIGURE 3.8. Budget-Constrained Total Utility (hedonic + Health).
[The IAPS] The food choice that maximizes total utility (hedonic + Health) is not necessarily the recommended level. The budget-constrained food choice matches the recommended level only when the budget is constraining and at the recommended level.

---

[2] To simplify the graph, we are only showing the decreasing marginal product and utility parts. Given the budget constraint locations, any other segments are irrelevant and therefore nothing is lost by excluding them.

and is added to the hedonic component to yield $h(F_1) + \beta H(F_1)$. Up until the recommended level F_1^R, everything is fine, as health utility *and* hedonic utility are increasing. However, beyond F_1^R, health utility begins to decline, so the individual is confronted with a tradeoff between health and hedonic utility: every additional bite or gram adds to his or her hedonic utility but subtracts from his or her health utility. The person will continue to consume more as long as the hedonic utility gain outweighs the health utility loss.

The point where the additional hedonic gain is offset by the health utility loss is then where their total utility, $h(F_1) + \beta H(F_1)$, is maximized, at F_1^T. This indicates that the total utility function, which incorporates the hedonic and health components, reaches a maximum at some level of consumption between the optimal health and optimal hedonic consumption levels. Stated more simply, the consumer reaches a compromise between hedonic utility and health utility. That makes sense, right?

What about income? At the low income (M^L/P_1) you cannot reach any of the optimal food levels: health (F_1^R), hedonic (F_1^h), or total (F_1^T). Income is binding. At the high income (M^H/P_1) you have enough income to reach the optimal health food level (F_1^R) but not enough to reach the optimal hedonic food level (F_1^h), *ignoring health*. However, you do have enough money to eat the amount of food that maximizes your *total* satisfaction at F_1^T. So, ultimately, *what determines the final optimal choice is how the budget constrains the combined or total utility, not the hedonic utility or health utility in isolation.*

The generality and usefulness of Figure 3.8 should be appreciated. It is not a static conceptual graph. In this example health utility reaches a maximum before the hedonic utility (e.g., a juicy fat tasty hamburger that is high in saturated fat). However, with some relabeling, the same figure can be modified to show when the hedonic utility reaches a maximum before the health utility, such as perhaps with vegetables. The general conclusion to draw from Figure 3.8 is that there are different levels of food consumption that are associated with optimal health, optimal unconstrained total utility, and optimal budget-constrained total utility. Figure 3.8 could therefore be labeled a *compromise graph*, because it shows how tradeoffs between competing objectives are integrated and reconciled. We will encounter compromise graphs later in the book as well.

Intellect-Enhancing Inquiries

1. Using Figure 3.8, explain how increasing the food budget may or may not lead to consumption closer to the recommended level.
2. Looking at Figure 3.8, think of examples of foods where health utility probably maximizes *before* hedonic utility (i.e., we eat too much) and examples of foods where health utility maximizes *after* hedonic utility (i.e., we eat too little).
3. Some people place a lot of emphasis on health utility and others place very little significance on health utility. Show and explain what would happen to Figure 3.8, and the implications for consumption, if an individual placed less significance on health utility (i.e., β decreases). What about more?

Conclusions

Congratulations. Your diligence has paid off. You now possess the main foundations required for the rest of this section of the book. Figure 3.8 is probably the most complicated figure in the entire book, so if you understand how to read it, you are on the verge of being fluent in the graphical language. With this solid foundation, let's continue the journey by looking at the more realistic case of more than one food in the next chapter.

Closing Conversation

JP: Thanks, Margaret. I can see why economics is a useful framework because it is quite general and integrates objectives, preferences, and constraints or barriers as we call them. As you pointed out, this seems overly simplistic. It does not allow for substitution, which seems important. Can you explain how the economic approach handles substitution?

Margaret: Delighted, but not now. I have to run. Can we continue this conversation tomorrow over lunch?

JP: Sure. I'll meet you at the Bag O Lunch shop at noon.

Margaret: Great. I look forward to it.

4

Income and the Importance of Substitution

Learning Objectives

What you will know by the end of this chapter:

¤ why substitution is so important in economics and nutrition;
¤ how to incorporate substitution in the analysis from Chapter 3;
¤ how to use the framework to analyze the expected impacts of a change in income or an income-targeted policy;
¤ the relationship between food and income as captured by the Engle curve; and
¤ some of the empirical findings relating income to food and nutrition choices.

Opening Conversation

JP: Hi, Margaret. A new hairstyle?
Margaret: Uh, yeah. So anyway, about substitution in economic analysis. We handle it this way.
JP: Oh, alright.

Why Is Substitution Important?

Economics is about choices. Choices involve weighing tradeoffs: Order a personal pizza or the chicken salad? Buy the Mercedes Benz or the Maserati? Date Sam or Mel? To solidify concepts, Chapter 3 considered only one food and one nutrient, so there was no substituting one food for another food. *Substitution* is the ability to buy one good in the place of another. Substitution is a critical concept in nutrition because food and nutrient recommendations can be met by many different combinations of foods and nutrients.

There are literally thousands of foods in the marketplace. However, the fundamental concepts can be captured with two foods and one nutrient. The components of the two-foods-and-one-nutrient model are the same as in Chapter 3. Given that income is the main limiting factor, we begin with the budget constraint.

The Food–Budget Relationship

Let's start with a simple example. Once a month, Mark joins his fellow graduate students for pizza and beer. Mark is in his late 20s and a stout guy of about 200 pounds. He recalls, from vaguely memorable but highly impressionable experiences, that his physical limit is a maximum of four beers or four slices of pizza. Of course, he could choose any combination: four beers + zero slices, two beers + two slices, three beers + one slice, and so forth. Suppose he is on a tight budget (welcome to graduate school!) and can afford to spend only $12. A slice of pizza costs $3 and a beer is also $3. So the question becomes, what is possible versus what is financially feasible? The total number of *possible* combinations is 25 (i.e., all combinations of zero up to four beers and zero up to four pizza slices), but several of these combinations will exceed his budget. For example, if he is completely parched, he could drink four beers (=$12) but eat no pizza. Alternatively, if he is really hungry and not thirsty, he could eat four slices of pizza (=$12) and drink no beer.

Figure 4.1 gives all the possible combinations as represented by the dots. However, Mark cannot afford anything above the line running from four pizza slices to four beers. For example, he can afford three pizza slices ($9) and one beer ($3)—point A. He can afford one pizza slice ($3) and three beers ($9)—point B. However, he cannot afford point C—three pizza slices ($9) and three beers ($9). Alternatively, if he buys one beer ($3) and one pizza slice ($3)—point D—he has $6 left over. So this line defines his feasible choice set. The *feasible choice set* is the set of all choice alternatives that are affordable given the budget constraint.

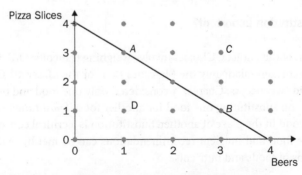

FIGURE 4.1. Unconstrained and Budget-Constrained Pizza and Beer Choices.

OK, let's generalize the above example. Suppose there are two food items, F_1 and F_2, such as beer and pizza slices, but it could be two food groups like protein foods and dairy. The prices of these two foods are denoted by P_1 and P_2. The budget constraint is the same as in Chapter 3 except we add the second food,

$$M = P_1F_1 + P_2F_2. \text{ Food - Budget Relationship} \tag{4.1}$$

Similar to Chapter 3, solve this equation for F_2 to yield

$$F_2 = \frac{M}{P_2} - \frac{P_1}{P_2}F_1. \text{ Isocost Line for Two Foods} \tag{4.2}$$

Equation 4.2 is called the *isocost line*. The term "iso" is Greek meaning equal. An isocost line is derived from the budget constraint and shows the tradeoff between the consumption of goods holding the budget or cost constant. This is simply the equation for a line with an intercept (M/P_2) and slope $(- P_1/P_2)$. The slope is especially important as it gives the opportunity cost of choosing one more unit of F_1. The term *opportunity cost* is a central concept in economics and is the cost associated with the forgone alternative or choice. It is what you give up for the choice you made. Using the numbers from the above example, $M = \$12$, $P_2 = \$3$, and $P_1 = \$3$, the isocost line is then $F_2 = 4 - 1.00\ F_1$. Choose the number of beers, F_1, you want, substitute this into the equation, and then you get the number of pizza slices you can afford, given your budget and the prices. The opportunity cost of one more beer is one less slice of pizza. Figure 4.2 gives the generalization of Figure 4.1.

Note a few key points from this graph:

◻ The isocost line exactly satisfies the budget constraint. Any point *on* the isocost line completely exhausts the entire budget. Along the isocost line are the substitution possibilities that all cost the same total amount.

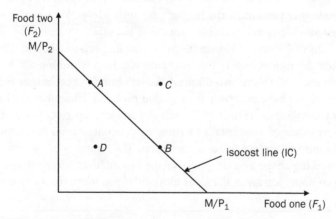

FIGURE 4.2. Isocost Line for Two Foods.
[The IAPS] Different combinations of two foods can have the same cost.

◻ The triangle defined by the isocost line is called the *feasible choice set.* Given the budget, any choice *outside* of the feasible choice set is unaffordable, such as C. Any choice *within* the feasible choice set is affordable, such as D, but does not use all of the budget.

◻ If the budget *increases,* the isocost line shifts *up* in a parallel fashion and the feasible choice set expands. More money means more feasible choices.

The Food–Preference Relationship

Within the feasible choice set, *any* combination of the two foods can be consumed. What combination will be chosen? Well, that depends on what an individual likes—his or her preferences or utility function. Just add the second food to the utility function.

Let's start just with the hedonic (only) utility function, which is now written as

$$U = h(F_1, F_2). \text{ Hedonic Food-Preference Relationship with Two Foods} \qquad (4.3)$$
$$\underset{(\pm)\ (\pm)}{}$$

The math paragraph (4.3) states that hedonic utility depends on how much of Food 1, F_1, and Food 2, F_2 (e.g., beer and pizza), are consumed. Utility is increasing and then decreasing for both food items (i.e., you like both of these items up to a point). So, we now have a relationship between three variables: the utility level (U), quantity of Food 1 (F_1), and quantity of Food 2 (F_2). However, we also have a problem. Three variables will correspond to three dimensions, but a piece of paper is two-dimensional. We must somehow show the relationship between three variables on a two-dimensional piece of paper. No problem.

Do you like to hike? A hiking analogy is perhaps the easiest way to see how the optimal choice will be made with two foods and represent this choice in two dimensions. Think of the utility function as a mountain that you want to climb. The higher you climb, the higher your utility level. Your goal is to get to the highest altitude (level) possible. You climb the utility mountain by choosing combinations of F_1 and F_2.[1] However, the isocost line acts as a barrier, like a wall built across the mountainside that prevents you from climbing all the way to the top. To show all this in two dimensions, let's borrow a technique from contour maps. If you have ever been hiking, you probably remember the logic of a contour or topographic (aka "topo") map. A contour map gives you a bird's-eye (from above) view of a mountain by showing concentric lines or contours. The contours represent points of equal elevation. The contours are useful because they tell you the shape and steepness of the mountain. As long as you stay on the same contour, you are at the same altitude. If you move from one contour to

---

[1] The online math supplement at http://www.aaec.vt.edu/people/faculty/davis-george.html has a fuller demonstration and discussion of this idea.

another, you change altitude. So we simply superimpose three utility contours over the isocost diagram as shown in Figure 4.3. Ignore the nutrient constraint for the moment.

How do you read Figure 4.3? Let's begin this hike by starting at point D, and remember that this is an aerial view. Think of the food quantities F_1^L and F_2^L as the longitude and latitude locations of point D, respectively. The low utility curve contour U^L shows the altitude associated with point D on the graph. The low income level is represented by the isocost line IC^L, which would look like the top of a wall from this aerial view, and prevents us from going any higher up the mountain. Now, suppose income increased. The increase in income M would cause the isocost line to shift up in a parallel fashion because both the x and y intercepts would be greater. The wall would be farther up the mountain.

Given that our goal is to get to the highest point on the mountain, we want to move to a higher utility contour. Shown in the figure are two higher utility contours: intermediate and high.

We could "walk" only east by consuming more of Food 1 and not changing Food 2 consumption until we got to point B, where we would hit the wall for high income. Alternatively, we could have walked only north and increased consumption of Food 2 only until we got to point A. However, points A and B are on the same utility contour, so they are at the same elevation and thus provide the same utility level. Consequently, the individual is indifferent between points A and B. This leads to the idea of an indifference curve. An *indifference curve* shows all combinations of goods that provide the same level of utility. The slope of the indifference curve measures the rate at which the individual would give up one good to get more of the other good without changing the utility level. This is called the *marginal rate of substitution.*

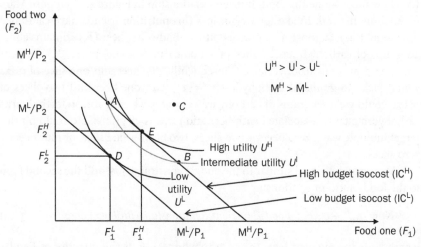

FIGURE 4.3. Budget-Constrained Utility Maximization with Two Foods and Two Income Levels. [The IAPS]As the budget increases, consumption of at least one food increases.

Can we do better than point *A* or *B*? Yes. While it is true the isocost line (the wall) associated with the higher budget level prevents us from going any farther east or north, remember that *any* point on the isocost line is feasible. All combinations along the isocost line cost the same amount. Consequently, by simply rearranging the combination of F_1 and F_2 (e.g., beer and pizza) we can reach a higher utility level (U^H) at point *E*—the combination of F_1^H and F_2^H. More generally, *the highest utility level will always occur where the indifference curve is tangent to the isocost line.* Think about it this way. If the vertical axis represents pizza consumption and the horizontal axis represents beer consumption, then this individual point *A* implies they are consuming too many pizzas and not enough beer for the amount of money they are spending. They would get more satisfaction spending the same amount of money by consuming fewer pizzas and more beer (i.e., moving toward point *E*). With the higher income level, similar arguments can be made for the other nonoptimal points *B* and *D*. Of course point *C* is still not feasible. Figure 4.3 is one of the most useful figures in the book and is just the two-food extension to Figure 3.7 from Chapter 3.

Dendrites Detour

1. In Figure 4.3, what would have to occur for the *intermediate* utility level to be the highest that could be reached? What would this imply for point *E*?
2. Under the above scenario, would the combinations *A* or *B* be chosen? Why or why not?

The Food–Nutrient Relationship

Let's now incorporate the food–nutrient relationship in Figure 4.3. Suppose Mark is watching his carb intake for weight loss (his nutrition friends have cautioned him about this). Suppose a 12-ounce bottle of Budweiser beer (F_1) contains about 12 grams of carbohydrates. A slice of a Pizza Hut Supreme pizza (F_2) contains about 24 grams of carbohydrates. Consequently, one beer and one slice of pizza would yield 36 grams of carbohydrates (=12 + 24), one beer and two slices of pizza would yield 60 grams of carbohydrates (=12 + 24 × 2), and so forth. Mark's carbohydrate target associated with beer and pizza is 48 grams. He could hit this target multiple ways: zero beers + two slices, two beers + one slice, or four beers + zero slices.

More generally, and similar to the budget constraint, just add the second food to the food–nutrient relationship as

$$N_1 = \alpha_{11}F_1 + \alpha_{12}F_2 : \textit{Food - Nutrient Relationship with Two Foods} \qquad (4.4)$$

where N_1 is the nutrient level (e.g., carbohydrates), F_1 is the quantity of Food 1 (e.g., beer), F_2 is the quantity of Food 2 (e.g., pizza), and α_{11} and α_{12} are the nutrient conversion factors for the two foods (e.g., 12 and 24).

To determine the substitution possibilities holding the nutrient intake constant, solve Equation 4.4 for F_2,

$$F_2 = \frac{N_1}{\alpha_{12}} - \frac{\alpha_{11}}{\alpha_{12}} F_1. \; \textit{Isonutrient Line for Two Foods} \tag{4.5}$$

Equation (4.5) is the *isonutrient line* and shows the tradeoff between the consumption of foods holding nutrient intake constant. Conceptually, it is very similar to the isocost line. If the nutrient level (N_1) increases or decreases, then the intercept (N_1/α_{12}) increases/decreases. The slope of the isonutrient line ($-\alpha_{11}/\alpha_{12}$) shows the nutrient opportunity cost of substituting one food for another. Because the "y and x" variables in the isocost and isonutrient lines are the same, we can just add the isocost line to Figure 4.3, as shown in Figure 4.4.

Let's first make sure the recommended isonutrient line (IN^R) is understood. Any combination of foods lying *below* the recommended isonutrient line means the recommended amount is not met. Any combination of foods lying *above* the recommended isonutrient line means the recommended amount is exceeded. But remember, *a nutrient recommendation is not binding!* Mark can afford to buy three pizza slices and one beer. If he decided to ignore his carbohydrate target of 48 grams and ate three pizza slices and one beer, he will consume 84 grams of carbohydrates ($3 \times 24 + 1 \times 12$). So, what will this mean in terms of translating the story of Figure 4.4 into words?

Given this individual's preferences and budget constraint, at the low budget level, point D is optimal (the tangency point). Yet, point D lies below the recommended isonutrient line, so he is below the recommended nutrient intake. To meet

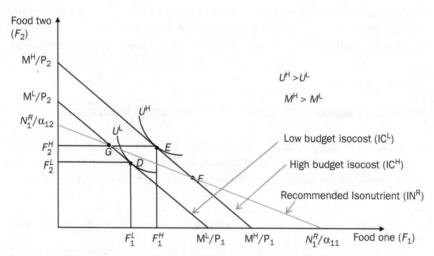

FIGURE 4.4. Budget-Constrained Utility Maximization with Two Foods, Two Income Levels, and Recommended Nutrient Intake.
[The IAPS]An increase in the budget may lead to a consumption bundle that exceeds the nutrient recommendations.

the recommended nutrient target, his preferences would have to be different such that his indifference curve would be tangent at point G. However, without different preferences, as his income increases, the new optimal consumption bundle will be at point E (the tangency point). Now he is exceeding the recommended nutrient intake, because point E is beyond the isonutrient line. Similar to point G, he would have to have different preferences for point F, the exact nutrient recommendation amount, to be optimal. In a nutshell, increasing income allows this person to meet and exceed the recommended nutrient level given his new income and preferences. One figure to help explain how increasing income can lead to multiple consumption patterns related to nutrient targets.

A Quickie

1. The slope of the isonutrient line is determined by how much of the nutrient is in each food (i.e., the nutrient conversion coefficients, the αs). Using Figure 4.4, show how to reach the nutrient target by consuming a different food with a higher nutrient content even at the low budget isocost line. What does this imply about needing more money to reach the nutrient target?

The (Nutrient) Food—Health Relationship

Are you wondering about the health component? Good. Proceed as with the other two relationships, but just add the second food to the health production function.

$$H = H(F_1, F_2): \; Food \text{-} Health \; Relationship \; with \; Two \; Foods \qquad (4.6)$$
$$\overset{(\pm)\;(\pm)}{}$$

As there are now multiple combinations of F_1 and F_2 that can lead to the same nutrient level, there are then multiple combinations of F_1 and F_2 that can lead to the same health level. As before, the little positive and negative signs indicate health is increasing and then decreasing in both F_1 and F_2.

Putting It All Together with Nutrient Recommendation Implications

We could write out the total utility function consisting of the hedonic utility (Equation 4.3) and health utility (Equation 4.6) in mathematical form as we did in Chapter 3, but the main insights come from the graph, so let's cut to the chase.[2]

---

[2] If you like the math, here is what the additive total utility function with two foods would look like:

$$U(F_1, F_2) \equiv h(F_1, F_2) + \beta H(F_1, F_2).$$
$$\overset{(\pm)\,(\pm)\quad\;\;(\pm)\,(\pm)\qquad\;\;\;(\pm)\,(\pm)}{}$$

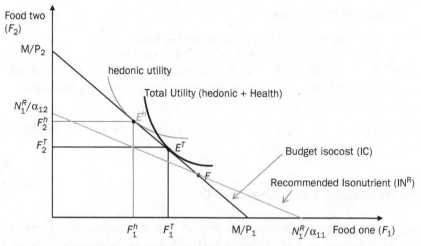

FIGURE 4.5. Budget-Constrained Total Utility (hedonic + Health) and hedonic-Only Maximization with Two Foods and Recommended Nutrient Intake.

[The IAPS]The food consumption that maximizes total satisfaction (hedonic + Health) and meets recommended intake does not necessarily maximize hedonic satisfaction alone.

Remember the key result from the compromise graph in Figure 3.8 with one food from Chapter 3: *what determines the final optimal choice is how the budget constrains the combined or total utility, not the hedonic or health utility in isolation.* This same concept applies with two foods. Figure 4.5 is the compromise graph for two foods.

For variety, let's change the two food items to be chicken sandwiches (F_1) and cheeseburgers (F_2) per month and the nutrient to fat intake. In terms of fat, the chicken sandwiches (F_1) have a lower fat content per gram and would be considered *relatively* healthier than the cheeseburgers (F_2). Given their budget constraint, when the individual pays attention only to hedonic utility (ignores health utility), the optimal consumption is $E^h \equiv (F_1^h, F_2^h)$.[3]

He is exceeding the nutrient requirement, represented by the isonutrient line IN^R (e.g., fat) because he is eating more cheeseburgers relative to chicken sandwiches.

However, when some importance is placed on the health utility, then the total utility indifference curve (hedonic + health) is the relevant indifference curve to consider and the optimal consumption combination is $E^T \equiv (F_1^T, F_2^T)$. The individual consumes fewer cheeseburgers and more chicken sandwiches. He is still over the fat target, but by considering the health effects of the foods, he is closer to the nutrient target than if he does not consider the health effects.

---

[3] You may be wondering why we don't also show the healthy utility curve in this graph as we did in Chapter 3, Figure 3.8. We don't really need it because the total utility indifference curve reflects the health utility as well. Because the total utility is a compromise between hedonic and health utility, the health utility indifference curve must be located to the southeast of the total utility indifference curve.

Check Your Competency

1. What happens to this graph if income increases?
2. What happens to this graph if the nutrient level increases?
3. What does the graph look like if the isocost and isonutrient lines do not intersect? (There are two possible cases). What are the implications of these two cases?

If you can answer these questions, you are crazy competent and well on your way to speaking economics fluently.

The Food–Income Relationship: Engel Curve

An *Engel curve* shows a direct relationship between income and the consumption of a good. Figures 4.4 and 4.5 can be used to derive the Engel curve as shown in Figure 4.6. Consider the top panel first. The optimal low income consumption bundle is $E^L \equiv (F_1^L, F_2^L)$. When income increases, the optimal high consumption bundle is $E^H \equiv (F_1^H, F_2^H)$, which is the tangency point with the higher total utility indifference curve. One can think of getting to this point in two steps. If only the hedonic utility is considered (health component is ignored), the individual would move to the optimal consumption at the tangency of the new isocost line and hedonic indifference curve $E^h \equiv (F_1^h, F_2^h)$. However, when some importance is placed on health, consumption is adjusted by consuming more of Food 1 and less of Food 2 until he reaches $E^H \equiv (F_1^H, F_2^H)$, which he considers to be the optimal compromise consumption satisfying both the hedonic and health utility.

The lower panel in Figure 4.6 shows the Food 1 Engel curve.[4] The horizontal axes on the upper and lower panels are both quantity of Food 1 (chicken sandwiches), so they can be connected. The lower panel vertical axis represents income. As explained above, as income increases, if the person pays attention only to hedonic utility, he will consume fewer chicken sandwiches than if he places some importance on health. This means the consumption of chicken sandwiches (Food 1) is *more* responsive to a change in income when health is taken into account than when it is ignored, as shown in the lower panel. Consistent with the upper panel, for this change in income and Engel curve, the change in income is still not enough to get to the recommended level F_1^R of this single food.

The responsiveness of consumption to a change in income is succinctly captured by the slope of the Engel curve: a flat Engel curve indicates greater responsiveness than a steep Engle curve. Note that the Engel curve is drawn as nonlinear (a non-constant slope) because it is believed that the responsiveness of consumption to a change in income is not constant and varies by preferences and levels of income.

---

[4] An Engel curve for Food 2 would be derived in exactly the same way.

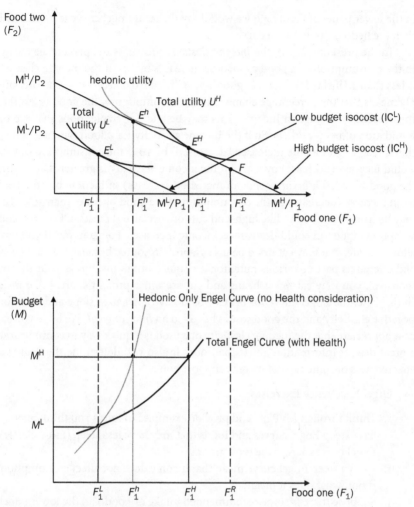

FIGURE 4.6. Utility Maximization and the Engel Curve with and Without Health-Effect Considerations for a Healthy Food.
[The IAPS]The relationship between income and food consumption (i.e., the Engel curve) varies with preferences.

Of course, different goods respond differently to changes in income. In economics, it is common to classify goods according to how they respond to a change in a variable, such as income, by an elasticity. *Elasticity* means the percentage change in one variable for a 1% change in another variable. As a good becomes more responsive to the change in another variable, we say it is becoming more elastic. Think of a rubber band and how elastic or stretchy it is. Some are more elastic than others. The same is true for goods, products, or variables. There are many types of elasticities—income, price, time—and they are generally characterized by their value relative to 1. If an elasticity is between 0 and 1 it called *inelastic*, if it is equal to 1 it called *unit elastic*, and if it is greater than 1 is called *elastic*. So in the lower panel of Figure 4.6 we would say the total Engel curve is more elastic than the hedonic-only Engle curve.

In the present context, the *income elasticity* measures the percentage change in the consumption of a good as income increases by 1%. If the income elasticity is less than 1 (inelastic), then the good is usually called a *necessity good*. This simply means that the percentage change in the consumption of the good is *less* than the percentage change in income. This may be true for staple foods that are the foundation of people's diets. So if the income elasticity for a food, say rice, is 0.25, this is read as "if income increased (decreased) by 10%, the consumption of food would increase (decrease) by 2.5%." If the income elasticity is greater than 1, then the good is called a *luxury good*: an increase (decrease) of income by 10% leads to an increase (decrease) in the consumption of the good by more than 10%. This may be true of something like high-end cuts or specialized meats. Of course, consumption of a good could *decrease* as income increases. For example, if you have a low income, you may eat dried beans as a protein source because they are cheap and offered as part of various nutrition assistance programs, but as your income increases, you may eat fewer beans and choose other protein sources like meat. In this case, the Engel curve for beans would have a negative slope and therefore negative elasticity and the good would be called an *inferior good*. We hope you can now appreciate that the income elasticity of a food is a quick way to communicate a great deal of information about that food. It also will determine the degree of effectiveness of some type of income support policy.[5]

Engel Excellence Exercises

1. Think through MyPlate and provide examples of foods you think may have steep Engel curves and foods that may have less steep (more elastic) Engel curves across the food groups.
2. Does a steep Engel curve mean that income does not affect consumption? If not, what does it mean?
3. Suppose there is some recommended intake of Food 1 in the lower panel of Figure 4.6. Will it be easier to reach the recommended level when income increases if the Engel curve is steep or flat?

Conclusions and Some Empirical Applications

We are all trying to optimize something (economists call it utility), but we are also trying to do this subject to constraints. There are usually numerous ways to meet the same objective, which implies there are substitution possibilities. In this chapter we have focused on substitution and demonstrated how this simple principle

---

[5] We have not shown the direct relationship between income and nutrition and income and health, but such relationships could be easily derived in a similar fashion. These would be called nutrient Engel curves and health Engel curves. Given the focus of this book, it all starts with food.

opens up many more possibilities in terms of meeting food and nutrient recommendations. Carrying over the income focus from Chapter 3, we turned toward deriving the Engel curve. The Engel curve shows the direct relationship between income and food consumption.

So what do we actually know about Engel curves? There is a very large literature looking at the relationship between income and food, income and nutrients, and income and health, and a review of this literature is beyond the focus of this book. However, we can give a few stylized facts:

- Food, nutrition, and health quality all appear to be positively related to income (Engel curves are upward-sloping), at least at a very aggregate level. Individuals with higher incomes generally consume more food · and have access to a wider variety of foods, consume foods with higher nutritional value, and have better health (e.g., Blisard, Stewart, and Jolliffe 2004; Darmon and Drewnowski 2008; Deaton 2002; Grimm et al. 2012; Hiza et al. 2013; Storey and Anderson 2014).
- People spend a smaller proportion of their income on food as their income rises, and Americans currently spend less than 10% of their money on food, the lowest in the world (U.S. Department of Agriculture, Economic Research Service, Food Expenditures 2014c).
- Engel curves and thus income elasticities vary a great deal and are moderated by numerous variables, such as education, socioeconomic status, geographic location, level of aggregation of foods, nutrients, and health indicators (e.g., Hiza et al. 2013; Storey and Anderson 2014). In the food recommendation context, where there is a lot of emphasis on understanding if an increase in income will improve diets via something like the Supplemental Nutrition Assistance Program (SNAP), the impact of income on improving diet *quality* appears to be rather small, at least for small changes in income (e.g., Blisard, Stewart, and Jolliffe 2004; Gregory et al. 2013). However, if the outcome of interest is food security (i.e., getting enough food) or general health, then several researchers have found that SNAP participation is associated with lower food insecurity and better health, although estimating the magnitude of the SNAP effect is quite challenging (e.g., Gregory and Deb 2015; Gundersen, Kreider and Pepper 2011; Li et al. 2014; Mabli and Ohls 2015).

As we move to the next chapter on prices, we will continue to use the two fundamental principles introduced in Chapters 3 and 4: optimization and substitution. Let the journey continue.

Closing Conversation

JP: Thanks, Margaret. The graphs are challenging, but the intuition is straightforward regarding tradeoffs and substitution. It is interesting how the analysis leads to a connection between income and food choices and that the Engel curve will vary by individual and by different foods. This helps explain the wide variety of effects across income-related programs, such as SNAP, and even other nutrition assistance programs like free and reduced school meal programs and WIC. However, there's something that's troubling about this analysis.

Margaret: Yeah, what is that?

JP: Well, you've assumed everyone faces constant prices. What if prices are different or change? What happens then?

Margaret: Well spotted, as my English friend Ken might say. Economics says a lot about prices, so you are right: we need to allow for prices to change in the analysis, but I have to go now. Can we continue this conversation over lunch tomorrow?

JP: I hear there is a new Thai restaurant on Maple Street. What about noon?

Margaret: Splendid. I look forward to it.

5

Prices

Learning Objectives

What you will know by the end of this chapter:

¤ why consumption increases as price declines—the law of demand;
¤ how responsive consumption is to price—price elasticities;
¤ how demand can increase without price decreasing; and
¤ what determines the ultimate effectiveness of food taxes or subsidies.

Opening Conversation

Margaret: Hey, JP! New haircut? I like it!

JP: Thanks. Sorry I'm late. I had to take my dog Blanco to the vet. So we were talking yesterday about how prices may affect food consumption. There has been a lot of discussion in the nutrition literature on the role of prices, such as blaming poor nutrition on the high price of healthy foods. Some have proposed taxes on unhealthy foods and beverages to make them more expensive to improve nutrition.

Margaret: I have a dog, too. Her name is Honey. Those are great applied economic issues. Should we order first? I am going to have the pad Thai. What would you like?

JP: Are you buying?

Margaret: Uh, sure, if you'd like.

JP: No, I was just kidding. I'll have the same thing.

Margaret: OK. Let's get back to your question. How consumption changes based on price depends on a lot of factors. The framework for income can be used for prices too, so let's go back there.

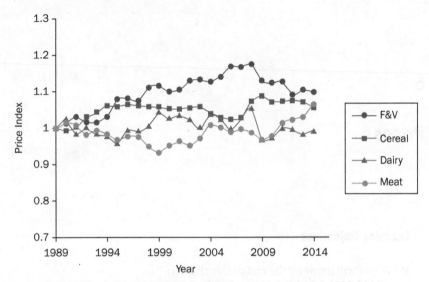

FIGURE 5.1 Real Price Indices of Some Major Food Groups (United States, 1989-2014).

Source: Bureau of Labor Statistics 2014. Relative to general food price index and base year 1989 equal to 1. F&V, fruits and vegetables; Cereal, cereals and bakery products; Dairy, dairy and related products; Meat, meat, poultry, fish, and eggs.

Some Data on Food Prices

As discussed in Chapter 2, average per capita U.S. consumption is below the recommended levels for fruits and vegetables, milk-related products, and whole grains. In contrast, consumption exceeds the recommended levels in refined grains, protein, saturated fat, added sugars, and sodium (U.S. Department of Health and Human Services 2010; Wells and Buzby USDA 2008). Are high and low prices to blame for these consumption patterns?

Figure 5.1 shows the price indices, a sophisticated average across locations, for four common food groups over the last 25 years in the United States. The fruit and vegetable price has been consistently higher than the cereal price, which has been consistently higher than the dairy price, which until about 2009 was higher than the meat price.

So the high price hypothesis supports the shortfall in fruit and vegetable consumption and the low price hypothesis supports the overconsumption of meat-related nutrients but not the underconsumption of dairy products. Apparently this price argument requires some refinement.

The Economics of Price Changes

How do prices affect food consumption? Intuitively, as the price of a good goes up, fewer people buy the item and each person probably buys fewer items. While perhaps usually true, this is not always the case. There is an important caveat that needs to be clarified. If you have a firm handle on the material in Chapter 3, this chapter will be a breeze. Let's start by stating the law of demand and deriving the demand curve before concluding with the more general idea of a demand function.

THE DEMAND CURVE

The law of demand is perhaps the *crème de la crème* of economic laws. The *law of demand* states that as the price of a good decreases, the quantity demanded for the good will increase, *ceteris paribus*. This is your intuition. But what is usually omitted is that odd Latin phrase, *ceteris paribus*. That is the caveat. *Ceteris paribus* means "all else constant." While prominent in economics, *all* scientific inquiries and explanations use the *ceteris paribus* concept, at least implicitly, to conceptually isolate the effect of a single factor on the phenomenon of interest.[1] We can all think of situations where a higher price would not necessarily mean that less of a product is bought, but this is usually because some other factor has offset the higher price. The *ceteris paribus* condition is not satisfied. We first need to understand the price effect in isolation when *ceteris paribus* is satisfied before we can understand when it is *not* satisfied.

Recall from Chapter 3 that the budget constraint contained prices, but there we focused on the effects of changing the budget, holding the prices constant. Now we reverse the analysis. Here we focus on the effects of changing the price, holding the budget constant, at least initially. Figure 5.2 demonstrates this process and is similar to Figure 4.6 from Chapter 4.

Start with the top panel. For concreteness, consider the case where Food 1, F_1, represents vegetables and Food 2, F_2, represents dairy. Initially the price of vegetables is relatively high at P_1^H and the optimal consumption bundle of vegetables and dairy is E^{High} —where the isocost line is tangent to the total utility indifference curve, U^0. Notice that the "x intercept" is M / P_1^H . If the price of Food 1 (vegetables) decreases to a lower price p_1^L the "x intercept" will increase, because P_1 is in the denominator. The feasible choice set has now expanded. The individual can consume more of Food 1 (vegetables) *and* Food 2 (dairy).

The individual can now move to a higher point on the utility mountain by changing the consumption bundle. If he focused only on the hedonic component of consumption—ignoring health effects—he would move to E^h, where the consumption of dairy (F_2) increased more than the consumption of vegetables (F_1). The amount of money he is now saving from a lower price of vegetables, P_1, is being used to purchase some more vegetables but mainly to purchase more dairy. However, if he takes into account the health effects (total utility), the optimal consumption bundle is E^{Low}. Relative to the hedonic-only point, E^H, at point E^{Low} there is now more consumption of Food 1 (vegetables) and less of Food 2 (dairy).

---

[1] See methodology appendix for more discussion.

What does a decrease in the price of vegetables (Food 1) mean for reaching some nutrient recommendation? The top panel includes a recommended isonutrient line (IN^R). Suppose the nutrient of interest is calcium. In general, dairy will have more calcium per gram than vegetables. If the individual just maximizes hedonic utility at E^h, he will be consuming too much dairy and calcium (i.e., above the recommended calcium intake). However, the recommended calcium level can be met by consuming less dairy and more vegetables at E^{Low}. At E^{Low} the actual and recommended vegetable intake will be equal (i.e., $F_1^1 = F_1^R$).

The lower panel in Figure 5.2 shows the demand curve for vegetables (F_1, Food 1). The lower and upper panels have the same horizontal axis. The lower panel's vertical axis is the price of vegetables (P_1, Food 1). As the price of vegetables, P_1, decreases and the individual completely *ignores* the health

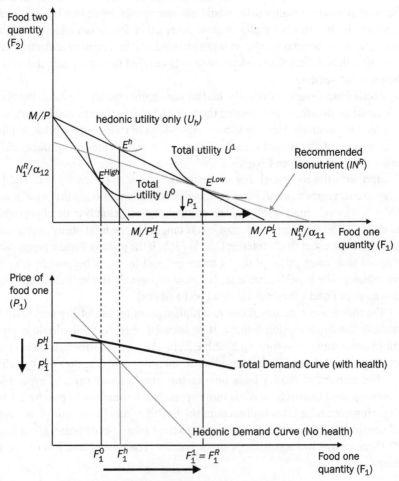

FIGURE 5.2 The Demand for a Food with and Without Health Considerations.
[IAPS]The Law of Demand: As price decreases, consumption increases, *ceteris paribus*—a movement *along* the demand curve.

utility component (hedonic only), he will increase his consumption of Food 1 (vegetables) only to F_1^h. However, if the health effects of vegetables are considered, the new consumption level will be higher at $F_1^1 = F_1^R$. Consequently, the lower panel captures the negative relationship between the price of a good and the quantity demanded for that good, *ceteris paribus*, which is the law of demand. The line drawn in the lower panel of Figure 5.2 is called the *demand curve*.[2] Each point on the demand curve gives the *quantity demanded* (e.g., 20 grams of vegetables) for the corresponding price. In addition, each price on a demand curve represents the *maximum* a consumer is willing and able to pay for the corresponding quantity. The collection of all the price and quantity-demanded combinations is called *demand* and is represented by the demand curve. A movement along the demand curve is a *change in quantity demanded*.

The slope of the demand curve, or more generally the demand elasticity, measures the change in the quantity demanded for a change in price. As we discussed in Chapter 4, an elasticity measures the percentage change in one variable as another variable changes by 1%. The *own-price demand elasticity* is the percentage change in the consumption of a good as the price of that same good changes by 1%. If the own-price elasticity is less than −1 it is called (own) *price elastic*, −1 *unit price elastic*, and between −1 and 0 *price inelastic*. As the hedonic demand curve is less responsive to a change in the price than the total demand curve (in this graph), it is more inelastic than the total demand curve.

As preferences differ by individuals, demand curves, and therefore elasticities, will also vary by individuals, but they will also vary by products. For example, perhaps your own-price elasticity for Granny Smith apples is −3, an elastic demand: a 10% increase in price leads to a 30% decrease in quantity demanded—a very high response to the change in price. Or your own-price elasticity of, say, locally grown strawberries may be −0.5, an inelastic demand: a 10% increase in price decreases quantity demanded by only 5%—a rather small response to the change in price. Because taxes or subsidies are designed to change prices, the effectiveness of food taxes and subsidies depends on the elasticities of demand.

Brain Breeze

1. Make a list of goods, not necessarily foods, you think may have elastic demands and a list that may have inelastic demands. Give your rationale. (Hint: Think extremes like cotton candy versus heroin.)
2. Repeat number 1 for foods, Is this more difficult? Why or why not?
3. If the own-price elasticity for sugar-sweetened beverages is −0.80 and a soft drink tax increases the price by 5%, soft drink consumption is expected to decrease by what percentage, *ceteris paribus*? If the target reduction in soft drink consumption is 10%, how much must the tax increase price?

---

[2] If it is called a demand curve, why is it drawn as a line? This a simplifying convention in economics. The most relevant fact is that it is negatively sloped, not that the slope can vary. Demand curves may be nonlinear or actual curves, but that added complexity is not central to the main points.

4. Consider these two statements:

"Taxes on sugar-sweetened beverages will reduce their consumption and therefore caloric intake."

"Taxes on sugar-sweetened beverages are not an effective instrument for reducing caloric intake."

Evaluate these two statements conceptually in terms of the elasticity of demand. Is one right and the other wrong, or are they both right or both wrong?

SHIFTS IN THE DEMAND CURVE

From Chapter 3 we considered the relationship between income and consumption, holding prices constant, and now we consider the relationship between own price and consumption, holding income constant. What if both changed? Someone may simultaneously face a reduction in income (being laid off) and an increase in the price of meat at the grocery store. Our framework would not be internally consistent or very useful if it were not able to handle such cases. Consequently, in this section we will consider what effects changes in income and the price of other foods will have on the demand for a food.

As seen in Figure 5.2, the horizontal axis for a demand curve will be the quantity of the food consumed (e.g., grams of vegetables). If an increase in *income* causes vegetable consumption to increase, holding price constant, then this increase must also show up on the demand curve graph for logical consistency. This is demonstrated in Figure 5.3. The top panel just repeats the Engel curve from Chapter 4. At the initial low budget M^L *and* some price P_1^0, consumption is F_1^L. As the budget increases to M^H, paying the same price per unit P_1^0, consumption increases to F_1^H. This change shows up in the lower panel as a *shift* in the demand curve to the right. If the demand curve did not shift to the right, we would have a logical inconsistency. The top panel would show consumption increasing on the horizontal axis as income increased, but the lower panel would show no change in consumption. How far will demand shift? The greater the income elasticity, the greater the demand shift. Of course, if income decreases, then the demand curve will shift to the left, for a normal good. So *a change in income causes a shift in the demand curve, not a movement along the demand curve.*

Let's consider another reason the demand curve may shift. To change it up a little, let's consider two different meats—chicken and steak. With a fixed budget for meat, if the price of steak increases, we would expect less steak and more chicken to be purchased. Figure 5.4 shows this case. The left panel shows the demand curve for steak (F_2). As the price of steak increases from a low price to a high price (P_2^L to P_2^H), the quantity demanded for steak decreases from F_2^0 to F_2^1. However, even though the price of chicken, P_1, did not change, because steak is now more expensive individuals substitute toward chicken. There is an increase in the demand for and consumption of chicken from F_1^0 to F_1^1 (right panel). So *a*

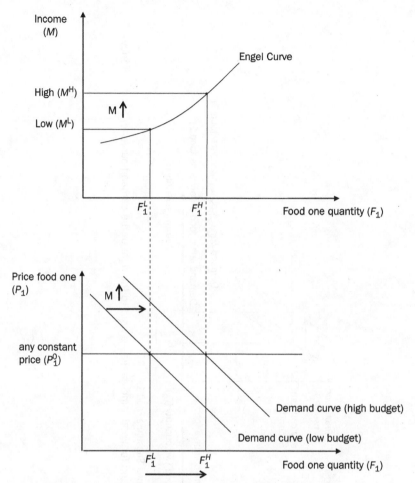

FIGURE 5.3 How Income Affects the Demand Curve for a Normal Good.
[IAPS] As income increases, demand for Food 1 increases—a *shift* to the right in the demand curve, for a normal good.

change in price of another good causes a shift in the demand curve, not a movement along the demand curve.

Figure 5.4 shows the case for two substitute goods. When an *increase* (*decrease*) in the price of one good causes an *increase* (*decrease*) in the demand for another good, the goods are called *substitutes*. Goods that are similar in many of their attributes are often substitutes. However, there are goods that are complementary, such as coffee and cream, or salsa and chips. When an *increase* (*decrease*) in the price of one good causes a *decrease* (*increase*) in the demand for another good, the goods are called *complements*. If the two foods in Figure 5.4 were complements, then the demand for Food 1 would shift to the *left* as the price of Food 2 increased.

How do we quantify these substitution effects across goods, as opposed to own-price effects? The same way we did for income and own price, with elasticities.

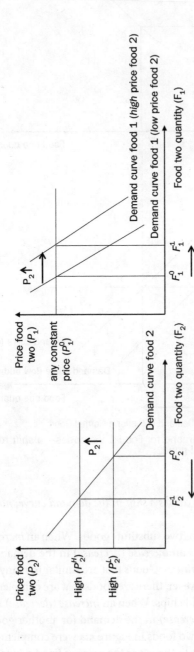

FIGURE 5.4 How the Price of Food 2 Affects the Demand for a Substitute Food 1.

[IAPS] As the price of Food 2 increases, the demand for Food 1 increases—a *shift* to the right of the demand curve for Food 1, if they are substitute foods.

A *cross-price demand elasticity* measures the percentage change in the quantity consumed of one good as the price of *another* good changes. For example, suppose the cross-price elasticity of chicken with respect to steak is 0.25. This means that for a 10% increase in the price of steak, the quantity demanded for chicken will increase by 2.5%.

Alternatively, if the cross-price elasticity of salsa with respect to chips is −0.50, then a 10% increase in the price of chips leads to a 5% decrease in the consumption of salsa. So a positive cross-price elasticity means goods are substitutes. A negative cross-price elasticity means goods are complements.

THE DEMAND CURVE VERSUS THE DEMAND FUNCTION

Are you starting to feel overwhelmed with the graphs? Are you wondering: *How do I remember all the variables and how they affect the demand for a food?* Here is a mnemonic device to help.

The figures used in Chapter 4 and here are powerful pictures and languages for communicating a great deal of information very quickly. If understood, they provide logical stories that disentangle the effects of intricate relationships in determining actual consumption. However, their main limitation is that they are two-dimensional. The vertical axis can show only one variable and the horizontal axis can show only another variable. Consequently, to show and tell the story, you must remember a graph for each relationship between two variables and you must remember what shifts the curve on that graph. There must be an easier way, right? Yes, there is. Just learn how to read and remember this:

$$F_1 = F_1(P_1, P_2, M, \varepsilon): \; \textit{Demand Function for a Food} \qquad (5.1)$$
$${\scriptstyle (-)\;(+)\;(+)\;(?)}$$

Trust us, it is easy. Read on.

Equation 5.1 is called a demand function and is the culmination of the individual maximizing his total utility when facing the budget constraint. The *demand function* is a multidimensional mathematical representation showing how multiple economic factors will affect the quantity demanded of a good, *ceteris paribus*. So how is this mathematics paragraph read in words? Like this. The quantity demanded for Food 1 (F_1), depends inversely on its own price (P_1), positively on the price of other (if a substitute) foods (P_2), positively on the budget (M), and in an unknown way with other factors (ε) not yet covered. The little negative, positive, or question symbols remind us of the direction of the relationships. Furthermore, the comma between all variables means these relationships are *ceteris paribus*.

But how does the demand function in Equation 5.1 help me in drawing graphs, you ask? Good question. As you read this paragraph, do the following—literally! Draw a horizontal axis and label it with the left-side variable F_1. Draw a vertical axis. Choose one of the right-side variables and place it on the vertical axis. Look at the little sign under the variable you chose. Draw a curve with a slope of the same direction as the sign. For example, suppose you chose the price of Food 1 (P_1) to place on the vertical axis. You then look at the little sign under P_1. You see it is negative, so you draw a negatively sloped curve. You have just drawn the demand curve for F_1. Alternatively, if you place budget (M) on the vertical axis and then draw the positively sloped curve as indicated by the sign, you have drawn the Engel curve.

But how does some *other* variable, *not* on the vertical axis, affect the curve you have drawn? Another good question. Look at the little sign under this *other* variable (e.g., P_2). If it is positive, this variable increases quantity demand, *ceteris paribus*, so an increase in this variable will shift the curve to the right. If the sign under the variable were negative, then an increase in this variable would shift the curve to the left. So, simply stated, the Engel curve and demand curve are two-dimensional representations of the demand function. The demand function is the unifying multidimensional concept underlying the Engel and demand curves.

Master Manipulator

1. Using Equation 5.1 as your guide, show what will happen to the Engel curve as the price of Food 1 increases. (Hint: With the same income, can you buy more or less of Food 1 if its price increases? This is just a reverse of which variables change in Fig. 5.3.)
2. Suppose you want to use the notation in Equation 5.1 to quickly summarize the demand for an inferior good, like Spam. What changes would you have to make to the notation? (Hint: If Spam is an inferior good, what happens to its consumption as income increases? How is that relationship shown in the Equation 5.1 notation?)

Conclusions and Empirical Applications

This chapter analyzed the effects of food prices on consumer choices using the foundational framework developed in Chapter 4. We presented the major components of neoclassical demand analysis: the law of demand, the demand curve, movements along a demand curve versus shifts in the demand curve, and an explanation of different types of elasticities. Two price-related areas have received a great deal of attention in the literature: comparative price analyses to determine if healthy foods are more expensive than unhealthy foods (e.g., Drewnowski and Darmon 2005; Drewnowski and Spectre 2004) and the effectiveness of using food taxes and subsidies to reduce weight (e.g., Brownell and Frieden 2009; Kim and Kawachi 2006).

There is a widely held view that "healthy" foods are more expensive than "unhealthy" foods, and there is now a rather large literature calculating and comparing the prices of different foods (for review see Rao et al. 2013). The evidence that healthy foods are more expensive than unhealthy foods is quite controversial. Some claim healthy foods are more expensive than unhealthy foods (e.g., Drewnowski and Darmon 2005), whereas others claim this is not the case (e.g., Carlson and Frazao 2012; Lipsky 2009). The general conclusion hinges on the units used in measuring prices, and three main units have been used: price per gram, price per serving, and price per kilocalorie. Only the price per kilocalorie shows "healthy" foods to be consistently more expensive (see Rao et al. 2013), but even this result is questionable as it apparently suffers from a fundamental analytical flaw (see, e.g., Davis and Carlson 2015; Lipsky 2009).

Of course, there is always the fallacy-of-composition problem: what is true of the total is not necessarily true of all its elements. Not all fruits and vegetables are more expensive (or less expensive) than all meats, even if expressed in the same units. Even for the exact same food item (e.g., strawberries), there is a great deal of variability in prices across space (e.g., region of the country), time (e.g., summer vs. winter), and form (e.g., frozen vs. fresh). These aggregation issues are exacerbated by trying to group together many different foods (pardon the pun, but apples and oranges). So, unqualified generalizations about prices are hard to come by.[3] Regardless, a higher price does *not* mean something cannot be afforded. Stewart et al. (2011) demonstrate that a variety of fruits and vegetables are actually affordable given prices, but consumers would have to change the mix of purchased foods. The problem is apparently more about preferences than prices.

Food and beverage taxes, and subsidies, have been proposed to help improve nutrition and consequently health (e.g., Brownell and Frieden 2009; Kim and Kawachi 2006). This literature has exploded in the last few years and there are now several good review articles (e.g., Andreyeva, Long, and Brownell 2010; Powell et al. 2013). In the context of this chapter, it should be clear that the effectiveness of food and beverage taxes or subsidies will depend on how responsive consumption is to changes in prices—the elasticity values. Andreyeva, Long, and Brownell (2010) provide the most comprehensive review across different food groups of elasticity values. Not surprisingly, there is variability within and across food groups and by study. However, on average for any food group, the own-price elasticity is always inelastic (i.e., between −1 and 0). As discussed earlier, the smaller the own-price elasticity, then the larger the price change and therefore tax or subsidy needs to be to get a large change in quantity consumed. For example, they find the average own-price elasticity for vegetables is −0.48. So if the target is to increase vegetable consumption by, say, 10%, then based on this elasticity value, the subsidy would have to decrease the price by 20%, *ceteris paribus*, which would require a very large subsidy.

On the tax side, sugar-sweetened beverages (SSBs) have received the most attention because they contribute the most calories and added sugars to consumption (Reedy and Krebs-Smith 2010). Powell et al. (2013) give a good summary of this literature and report that SSBs are more price-sensitive than other foods, with an average own-price elasticity of −1.21. This elastic own-price response suggests that an SSB tax may be an effective way to reduce calories. For example, if the price is increased by 10%, then consumption of SSBs should decrease by 12%,

---

[3] The subdiscipline of aggregation and index numbers in economics is designed to provide a theoretically sound and standardized basis for constructing aggregate prices that are comparable. Unfortunately, theoretically consistent food price indices are seldom encountered in the nutrition and public health literature, so the aggregation procedures fall victim to many of the limitations explained in the aggregation literature. There are some notable exceptions, such as Christian and Rashad (2009) or Powell and Bao (2009).

and therefore calories would decrease by 12%, right? Wrong! We are forgetting the importance of that little *ceteris paribus* caveat. Calories are determined by the consumption of *all* foods and beverages. As the SSB price increases, there will be changes in the consumption of other foods and beverages: substitution matters. Numerous studies have taken into account substitution effects, and the general finding is that substitution effects reduce the effect of an SSB tax on caloric intake (e.g., Dharmasena and Capps 2012; Finkelstein et al. 2013; Lin et al. 2011; Zhen et al. 2014).

Are we to conclude that price instruments like taxes or subsidies are not effective policies? No, they are just not the silver bullet of policy interventions to fight obesity (Block and Willet 2013). Taxes and subsidies are just one of many tools in the toolbox. Of course, the discussion and implementation of taxes and subsidies on certain foods do reflect social concerns and political priorities.

Let's pack our bags and move on to talk about the role of convenience in the next chapter.

Closing Conversation

JP: Thanks, Margaret. I can see that the economic framework is appealing because of its coherency. I am very curious about the answer to the Brain Breeze question #3 you posed on an SSB tax. Can we work through one together? That question says the own-price elasticity of SSBs is −0.80, and suppose the tax increased the price by 5%. What will the effect be? My answer would be given that the own-price elasticity measures the percentage change in consumption for a 1% change in price, then it just seems like a 5% change would be five times that, or 5 × −0.80, or −4%: a 4% decrease in the consumption of SSB. Is that right?

Margaret: You catch on quite quickly. Yes, that's right.

JP: Cool! So using this little elasticity relationship, if I want a 10% decrease in the consumption of SSBs, and given that the own-price elasticity measures the percentage change in consumption for a 1% change in price, I could take the quantity reduction of −10% and divide it by the own-price elasticity −0.80 to get 12.5% (=−10/−0.80). So if I wanted to decrease SSB consumption by 10%, I'd have to increase the price of SSBs by 12.5%. Correct?

Margaret: Very good—sort of.

JP: What do you mean, "sort of"? Is something wrong with my math?

Margaret: No, your math is fine. You are just forgetting the *ceteris paribus* assumption—all else being constant. If all else were constant, then your number would be a good estimate.

JP: I want to talk about this some more, but I have to go. I've got a time constraint. I'm curious what else may matter.

Margaret: OK—you just identified another possible factor!

JP: Huh? I've got to go. What about dinner tomorrow night?

Margaret: OK, let's say 7:00 at Desperado.

JP: Lovely. See you there.

6

Convenience and Time

Learning Objectives

What you will know by the end of this chapter:

¤ the recent patterns in food at home and food away from home expenditures and how these are related to employment patterns in the United States;
¤ how money *or* time may be the main constraint to healthy eating;
¤ the difference between the money price of a food and the full price of a food, and why that difference is important; and
¤ how changing the value of time changes the demand for food.

Opening Conversation

JP: Hey, Margaret. Our table will be ready in about 15 minutes. What is that in your hand?

Margaret: I bought your dog Blanco a little get-well toy.

JP: Thanks! That is very thoughtful. So we've talked about how changes in income may affect food choices and how changes in price may affect food choices, but surely there are other important factors. For example, on Tuesdays I volunteer at a local food bank and don't finish until about 8:00 p.m. After that I just want to order takeout; I don't want to cook. Price or income has not changed, so how does economics explain that decision?

Margaret: That is a very rational decision. Well, in this case the little Latin phrase *ceteris paribus* doesn't apply—all else is *not* the same. We need to add a time constraint and value of time into the analysis.

Background on Convenience and Food Expenditures

Convenience is the ease of acquiring a good or service with the goal of saving time and effort. Convenience is usually preferred to inconvenience and can occur in many forms: accessibility, extended store hours, online ordering, or self-service checkout. Indeed, "convenience" has emerged as a category in cookbooks, starting perhaps with Rachel Ray's *Thirty Minute Meals* (Ray 2006), only to be topped by Jamie Oliver's *Fifteen Minute Meals* (Oliver 2012). Convenience is a major factor in food choices. For example, Glanz et al. (1998) found that the four most important factors in determining food choices were (in descending order) taste, cost, nutrition, and convenience. We have already integrated taste (preferences), cost, and nutrition into a unified framework. Now we will add convenience. The key characteristic of a *convenience food* is that it is designed to save time and effort—to be labor-saving. This will usually involve some level of processing designed to save labor.[1]

A common way to partition convenience foods is by food at home (FAH) and food away from home (FAFH). FAH is food purchased from any food outlet except a restaurant—such as a grocery store, supermarket, farmers' market—for use in home food production. FAFH is food bought usually for immediate consumption from a food service provider, such as a restaurant, and would include food at schools.

Figure 6.1 shows how spending on FAFH has increased relative to FAH in the United States since 1982 (top line). This trend is not only of economic interest but also of public health interest because FAFH generally contains more calories, total fat, saturated fat, sugar-sweetened beverages, and sodium and lower levels of fruits, vegetables, and dairy compared to FAH (see review article by Lachat et al. 2012).

Furthermore, consuming more FAFH relative to FAH contributes to lower dietary quality and, as a result, higher risk for obesity (see review article by Bezerra et al. 2012). More directly, those spending more time in food preparation at home tend to have healthier diets (e.g., Monsivais, Aggarwal, and Drewnowski 2014).

So, what has been the main force (not the only one) behind this redistribution of total food expenditures towards FAFH? A strong case can be made that it is mostly related to time. Why? Over the last 30 years the women's labor force participation rate has increased relative to men's, as also shown in Figure 6.1 (bottom line). But women are still the primary gatekeepers of food and nutrition in households. As a result, less time is available for all aspects of food preparation (e.g., meal planning, grocery shopping, food preparation, cooking), therefore increasing the demand for convenience foods that require less time, *ceteris paribus*. Note the trends in FAFH relative to FAH expenditures and women's labor force participation rate (relative to men's) move in near unison.

---

[1] Poti et al. (2015) provide a good analysis and discussion of the distinction between processing level and convenience.

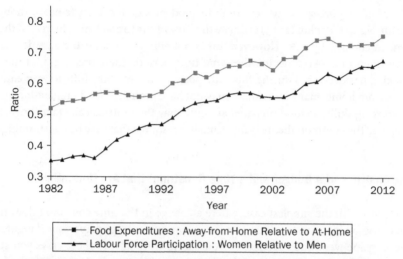

FIGURE 6.1 Food Expenditures and Labor Force Participation, Food Away from Home Relative to
Food at Home and Women's Labor Force Participation Rate Relative to Men, 1982–2012.

Source: U.S. Department of Agriculture. Economic Research Service 2014c and Bureau of Labor
Statistics. Employment. 2014. Authors created figure.

Figure 6.2 shows how much time was spent in food preparation at home by
employment status, gender, and engagement status in 2011. In this context engagement is not related to marriage; engagement means an individual reported spending some time in food production activities on the day he or she was surveyed.
"All" includes reported time in food production for both disengaged (no time) and
engaged (some time) individuals for the survey day. Not surprisingly, employed
individuals spend less time on food production activities than unemployed ones.

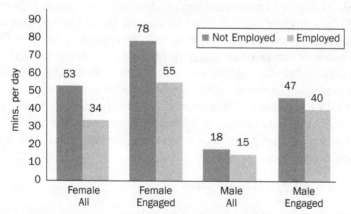

FIGURE 6.2 Minutes per Day in Food Production by Employment Status, Gender, and Engagement
in Food Production, 2011.

Engaged = those reporting positive time in food production.

Source: Bureau of Labor Statistics, American Time Use Survey, 2014. Authors' calculations.

Males report spending less time in food production than females, though Smith, Ng, and Popkin (2013) estimate that from 1965 to 2008, men increased their time in cooking by 13%. However, this is not enough to offset the 24% decrease by women in cooking during the same time period. Therefore, overall, time in cooking has decreased during this time period. Finally, with shifts toward eating away from home, many individuals may not have proficient food preparation and/or cooking skills, so food prepared at home may then intrinsically take longer to prepare. The common theme is that time is a resource that may be constraining.

The Analytics of a Budget and a Time Constraint that Are Unrelated

Let's start with the simplest case, where a change in the time constraint does not affect the budget constraint or vice versa. For example, perhaps your daughter's soccer game went into overtime or you had to work late. In these cases you still have the same amount of money, but less time. Alternatively, suppose you had to replace the transmission on your old car, so you have less money to spend on food. You still have the same amount of time, just less money. These are examples of where the budget and time constraint are unrelated.

For concreteness, let F_H represent the quantity of FAH and F_A the quantity of FAFH, with corresponding prices P_H and P_A. The budget constraint is as before:

$$M = P_H F_H + P_A F_A : \; Budget \; Constraint \tag{6.1}$$

Rearranging the budget constraint in Equation 6.1, we get the isocost line

$$F_H = \frac{M}{P_H} - \frac{P_A}{P_H} F_A : \; Isocost \; Line \tag{6.2}$$

The budget constraint captures the idea of a financial constraint and the financial tradeoffs the consumer faces. However, we can also think of a time constraint and each food item as having a "time price" as well. For example, if you go to Chipotle to eat a burrito, it may take 20 minutes to order and eat it. Alternatively, if you prepare a burrito at home, it may take 45 minutes to prepare and eat it. The logic for a time constraint is completely analogous to that of a budget constraint.

Let T be the amount of time deemed available for the two foods. The time prices for F_H and F_A are denoted as T_H and T_A, respectively. The *time price* is the amount of time it takes to produce or consume one unit of the item. The time constraint is written as

$$T = T_H F_H + T_A F_A : \; Time \; Constraint \tag{6.3}$$

The isotime line derived from Equation 6.3 is then

$$F_H = \frac{T}{T_H} - \frac{T_A}{T_H} F_A : \; Isotime \; Line \tag{6.4}$$

The slope of the isotime line gives the opportunity cost *in time* of consuming one more unit of F_A. For example, if it takes 60 minutes to make and eat a pizza at home ($60 = T_H$) but 30 minutes to eat a pizza out ($30 = T_A$), then the time opportunity cost of eating a pizza out is half of that at home (i.e., ½ = 30/60).

The isocost and isotime lines can be placed on the same graph as they both contain F_A and F_H (Fig. 6.3). Though this figure resembles the isocost–isonutrient figure from Chapter 4 (Fig. 4.4), there are some important differences stemming from the differences between the isonutrient line and the isotime line:

1. The *isonutrient line is not a binding constraint* that the individual *must* consume on or below. The individual can violate the isonutrient line in consuming food items.
2. The *isotime line is a binding constraint*, assuming that the isotime line represents all time available for the consumption of these two items. The individual cannot violate the isotime line in consuming food items. (We will consider in a few pages the case where the consumer can make choices that may change the isocost and isotime line.)
3. As a result of (1) and (2), the feasible choice set with a budget and time constraint is determined by the *intersection* of the budget feasible choice set and the time feasible choice set (the shaded quadrilateral area in Fig. 6.3).

The points in Figure 6.3 represent different combinations of F_A and F_H corresponding to different individuals (preferences) who all have the same time and budget constraint. The food combinations represented by points A_1, A_2, A_3, and A_4 all lie on the same *isotime line* (IT), so all cost the same amount of time and are

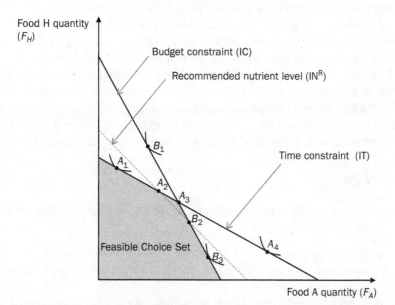

FIGURE 6.3 Feasible Choice Set and Optimal Consumption with a Budget and Time Constraint. [IAPS] Some lack income and some lack time, so nutrient recommendation may not be met for different reasons.

time-feasible. Similarly, the food combinations represented by points B_1, A_3, B_2, and B_3 all lie on the same *isocost line* (IC), so all cost the same amount of money and are money-feasible. What's the problem?

Consider an individual who prefers eating a high percentage of FAH, F_H, relative to FAFH, F_A. If there was *only* a budget constraint, then this individual would maximize utility at point B_1. However, because of the time constraint, the highest level of utility he can reach is at point A_1. Time is the binding constraint, not money. This individual is "money-rich" but "time-poor." Alternatively, consider a different individual who would like to maximize utility at point A_4. However, because of the budget constraint the highest level of utility he can reach is at point B_3. For this individual, money is the binding constraint, not time. He is "money-poor" and "time-rich." Thus the *feasible choice set* is determined by the intersection of the budget feasible choice set and the time feasible choice set. Recognize the different constraints are binding at different points because of different preferences (i.e., indifference curve locations).

What are the implications for meeting the nutrient recommendations? The nutrient recommendation level is represented with the isonutrient line (IN). The two individuals represented by A_1 and B_3 are below the recommended nutrient level but for different reasons. Individual A_1 falls short because he does not have enough time to support these preferences. Individual B_3 falls short because he does not have enough money to support these preferences. Note, however, both *could* reach the recommended nutrient target because any point lying on the line between points A_2 and B_2 is feasible and meets the recommendation. However, for individual A_1 it would involve allocating less *time* consuming FAH and more FAFH (i.e., a change in preferences). Alternatively, for individual B_3 it would involve allocating less *money* consuming FAFH and more FAH (i.e., a change in preferences).

Preferences can be hard to change, but the recommended nutrient may be reached alternatively by relaxing the time constraint as shown in Figure 6.4. As time allocated to these two foods increases, the *isotime* constraint shifts up, just like we saw with the budget constraint in Chapter 4. The feasible choice set is now expanded by the darker trapezoid area in Figure 6.4. The consumer now maximizes utility by consuming at point B_1, which will satisfy the nutrient recommendation, as it lies on the isonutrient line. While we have used the example of FAH and FAFH as the motivating example, it should be clear that the analysis generalizes to *any* two foods.

Time Out

Consider how the *slopes* and therefore the feasible choice set will change for the following cases:

- What happens to Figure 6.3 if the time price of food at home T_H decreased (e.g., you replace your conventional oven with a convection oven, which cooks faster)?
- What happens to Figure 6.3 if the money price of FAFH P_A increased (e.g., your favorite restaurant raised the prices on its menu)?

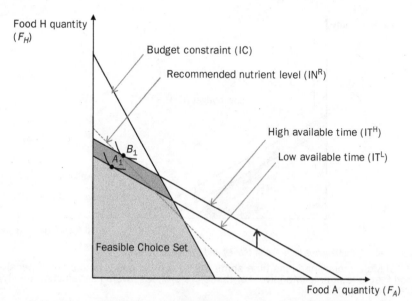

FIGURE 6.4 Feasible Choice Set and Optimal Consumption with an Increase in Time Budget. [IAPS] More time increases choice options, especially those that require more time, allowing the nutrient recommendations to be reached.

¤ What happens to Figure 6.3 if the amount of nutrients in FAFH α_{1A} decreased (e.g., saturated fat)?

The Analytics of a Budget and a Time Constraint that Are Related

There are many scenarios where money and time are related. The analytical approach is no different. Just proceed in steps, working with one constraint at a time.

Consider a specific example. Mellie was unemployed but now has a job. She now has *more money* but *less time* to spend on food, as shown in Figure 6.5. The original feasible choice set is defined by the light-gray area *and* the medium-gray area (i.e., low budget, high time).

Mellie was maximizing utility at point A with about an equal consumption of FAH (F_H) and FAFH (F_A). At this point, Mellie is time-rich but money-poor as the time constraint is not binding but the money constraint is binding. After getting a job, the new feasible choice set is now the light-gray area plus the dark-gray area. The medium-gray area was lost but the dark-gray area gained. The original consumption bundle at point A is no longer feasible, because there is not enough time. Mellie is now money-rich (high budget) but time-poor (low time), and the new optimal bundle is at point B, where she consumes more FAFH (F_A) and less FAH (F_H). The way this diagram is drawn, she is at the same utility level (on the same indifference curve) before and after the change. The key point is that increasing

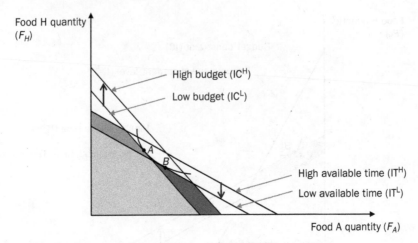

FIGURE 6.5 Simultaneous Increase in Money and Decrease in Time.
[IAPS] More money and less time shifts the choice options toward more expensive food that is less time-intensive. For these preferences, overall satisfaction (utility) does not change.

income and decreasing time does not necessarily mean she will be more satisfied (i.e., at a higher indifference curve).

Time Is Money: Converting the Time Constraint into Monetary Units

Figures 6.3 through 6.5 are very good for showing one can be money-rich and time-poor or vice versa, but they are rather unwieldy for showing changes in resources and prices. Is there a simpler way to incorporate time in the analysis? Well, yes. As Benjamin Franklin said, "Time is money." Time can be converted into a dollar value. You can think about this approach by answering this question: How much would you pay for a unit of time? For example, suppose you go to a popular restaurant without a reservation and there is a waiting line. An enterprising but unfair attendant asks how much you would pay to be seated immediately. You pause and then say $10. You have just revealed the monetary value of your time in waiting. This logic can be extended to almost any activity. We often pay more for some good or service not because we cannot do it ourselves, but because we value our time more than the extra money we would have to pay. By placing a monetary value on a unit of time, we can combine the budget and time constraints into the full cost constraint.

For each activity requiring a unit of time, let w_i be the *time cost conversion factor* that converts a unit of time into its dollar equivalent. This time conversion factor will be unique to each individual depending on how he or she values time spent in the activity.[2] Now, if an activity takes T_i units of time, then the *money time*

---

[2] A common approach taken in measuring this conversion factor is to assume that an individual's wage rate can be used to value an individual's time in *all* activities. This is true under certain assumptions and would be a special case of what is presented here.

price in this activity will be $w_i \times T_i$. For example, suppose that it takes 30 minutes to eat one meal at Outback and you value each minute at $0.10. The money time price for this one meal is then $w_i \times T_i = \$0.10 \times 30 = \$3$.

Let's now use this idea of the money time price to create the full cost constraint. The *full cost constraint* is the sum of the money food cost and the money time cost, or

Full Cost = Money Food Cost + Money Time Cost

Continuing the FAH (F_H) and FAFH (F_A) example, the full cost constraint can be written as

$$FC = (P_H F_H + P_A F_A) + (w_H T_H F_H + w_A T_A F_A). \tag{6.5}$$

The first parenthetical term is the budget constraint. The second parenthetical term is the time constraint expressed in money units. More insight comes from collecting like terms and rearranging Equation 6.5 to yield

$$FC = (P_H + w_H T_H)F_H + (P_A + w_A T_A)F_A : Full\ Cost\ Constraint \tag{6.6}$$

Equation 6.6 indicates that the *full price* of a food item is then the food price (P_i) plus the money time price ($w_i T_i$). The full price is an extremely useful construct because it allows one to consider obvious tradeoffs that can occur between money and time.

Here is an example of why distinguishing the *food price* from the *full price* of a food item is important. Suppose you are considering ordering a pizza for delivery or making one at home. The delivery pizza cost $12 and takes 5 minutes to order and 25 minutes for the pizza to be delivered. The ingredients for the pizza at home cost $6 and it takes you 120 minutes to prepare and bake it. You value the time for each pizza the same at $0.10 per minute. The relevant values are then $P_A = \$12$, $T_A = 30$, $w_A = \$0.10$, $P_H = \$6$, $T_H = 120$, and $w_H = \$0.10$. The full price of the delivery pizza is $P_A + w_A T_A = \$12 + \$0.10 (30) = \$15$, whereas the full price of the pizza at home is $P_H + w_H T_H = \$6 + \$0.10 (120) = \$18$. Note that ignoring the time cost component, the pizza at home appears to be the better bargain, costing half the amount as the restaurant pizza (i.e., $6 vs. $12). However, once we consider the time component as well, the full price of the pizza at home is $3 more than the pizza in the restaurant (i.e., $18 − $15 = $3). This example should appeal to your intuition and reveal the usefulness of this concept. How many times do you decide to eat somewhere not because the food cost is high, but because the time cost is high or vice versa?

How does all of this simplify Figures 6.3 through 6.5 as promised? Using the idea of a full price, we have basically converted a two-constraint problem to a single-constraint one. We can therefore use our normal isocost graph with a little relabeling. For notational ease and cognitive connection, let's use the symbol Π to denote the full price, so $\Pi_H = P_H + w_H T_H$ and $\Pi_A = P_A + w_A T_A$. Direct substitution into Equation 6.6 yields

$$FC = \Pi_H F_H + \Pi_A F_A \qquad (6.7)$$

Proceeding as before, just solve Equation 6.7 for the full isocost line, or

$$F_H = \frac{FC}{\Pi_H} - \frac{\Pi_A}{\Pi_H} F_A : \textit{Full isocost constraint} \qquad (6.8)$$

We are now back in business and can simply use all of the graphing devices from Chapter 5 with a little relabeling.

Figure 6.6 shows what would happen to changes in consumption of FAH (F_H) and FAFH (F_A) as the full price of FAH increased and how this is related to a nutrient target.

The *full feasible choice set* is the triangle defined by the full isocost line. Prior to the increase in the full price of FAH, Π_H, the individual was consuming a combination of FAH and FAFH that was maximizing utility *and* satisfying the nutrient requirement (i.e., point E^{low}). As the full price of FAH, Π_H, increases, the full isocost line rotates clockwise and the full feasible choice set shrinks away from FAH, F_H. The new optimal consumption bundle is now below the nutrient recommendations at E^{high}. So all the techniques you learned in Chapter 5 with the simple isocost line are applicable here except for one caveat: the full price and therefore the full isocost line slope can change for one of three reasons. Note that the full price in general is $\Pi_H = P_H + w_H T_H$, so it may change if (1) the food price, P_H, changes or (2) the money value of time spent on the food item w_H changes, or (3) the amount of time per unit of food item, T_H, changes.

Before concluding this section, we want to be clear on what the terms *full price* and *full cost* do and do not cover. An appealing feature of the economic approach is the precise and clear distinction that it makes between costs and benefits. For the individual, in the economic approach, costs correspond to the outlay of *personal* resources: How much of your money and time do you sacrifice in making a choice? Thus the terms *full price* and *full cost*, which come from Becker's (1965) seminal work, refer only to resource constraint-based prices and costs. Alternatively, benefits, in the economics of consumer choice, refer to the overall satisfaction (utility) the individual gets from the purchase or decision. With any choice there can be positive and/or negative benefits (utility) that have nothing to do with the individual's resources, such as cooking enjoyment, cultural acceptability, and environmental impact. These attributes affect utility but not available resources. People who enjoy cooking do not have a negative cost associated with cooking; rather, they have a positive utility. They still incur a cost of time, but this is offset to some degree by their enjoyment of cooking. A negative impact on the environment of a choice may be a "cost" in laymen's terms but is not considered a cost in the economic framework of individual choice. In the economic framework, a negative benefit is called *disutility*. So the terms *full price* and *full cost* need to be understood and used in the context of the personal resource constraint. These distinctions may seem like hair-splitting, but precision in language and terms is very important, especially when it comes to identifying effective policy interventions. Misclassifying something as a "cost" when it is actually an attribute that provides

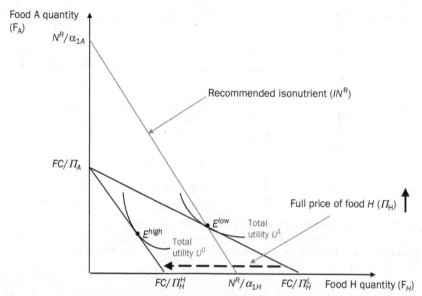

FIGURE 6.6 Change in the Feasible Choice Set with an Increase in the Full Price of Food H. [IAPS] As the full price of FAH, including money and time, increases, the feasible choice set shrinks away from FAH.

disutility (e.g., a bad ambiance for eating) may suggest that more money or time would fix the problem, when in fact money and time are not the issue.

The Full Monty

Can you do "the full Monty" with this graph (i.e., show all it can do)? Starting from an initial equilibrium in Figure 6.6 E^{high}, draw the appropriate graph for the following scenarios.

- Eric likes Mexican food. A new Chipotle, a Mexican fast casual dining restaurant, is built across the street from Eric's house.
- Sam and Brenda bought a new convection oven that reduces cooking time at home.
- Tony retires from his job. State any assumptions that are being made.

The Demand Curve and Time

As indicated in Chapter 5, demand is a fundamental concept in economics. Now that you have the foundations from Chapter 5 in place, we can use our mnemonic device of a demand function to quickly determine how time affects demand. As seen above, the only difference between what we did in Chapter 5 and here is we added a time constraint, T, and we redefined prices, P, to be full prices, Π. Consequently we could just modify Equation 5.1 from Chapter 5 accordingly as

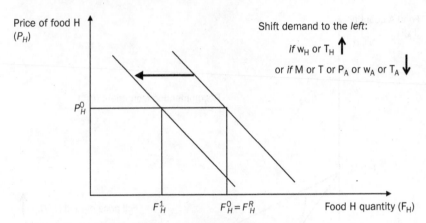

FIGURE 6.7 The Demand for a Food H and Demand Shifters.
[IAPS] The demand for Food H decreases if it takes more time to consume or the full price of a substitute food decreases, or there is less money or time.

$F_1 = F_1(\underset{(-)}{\Pi_1}, \underset{(+)}{\Pi_2}, \underset{(+)}{M}, \underset{(+)}{T}, \underset{(?)}{\varepsilon})$. This is not a great mnemonic device because we would still have to remember that each full price could change for the three reasons mentioned above. To make it completely transparent, substitute for each full price, $\Pi_i = P_i + w_i T_i$ to yield

$$F_1 = F_1(\underset{(-)}{P_1 + w_1 T_1}, \underset{(-)\ (-)}{P_2 + w_2 T_2}, \underset{(+)\ (+)}{M}, \underset{(+)}{T}, \underset{(?)}{\varepsilon}). \qquad (6.9)$$

All we have done is just added the w_i, T_i and T terms to the demand function from Chapter 5. To draw the demand curve, place the variable F_1 on the horizontal axis and its money price, P_1, on the vertical axis. The negative sign under P_1 indicates that you should draw a downward-sloping curve, and you have drawn the demand curve. All *other* variables are then demand *shifters*. Figure 6.7 shows the demand curve for Food 1. For example, if this were demand for FAH F_H, then anything that caused the full price of FAH to increase *other* than the money price of food P_H, such as the value of time (w_H) or the amount of time (T_H), would cause the demand for FAH to decrease. The individual may then be below some target recommendation level F_H^R. This should make sense. All else constant, if the time cost associated with a good increases, you will consume less of it. Changes in other variables are interpreted similarly.

Conclusions and Empirical Applications

Convenience is clearly an important attribute that is taken into account when buying and consuming food. The obvious unit for measuring convenience is time. Time is perhaps the ultimate constraint or barrier in life, and our economic framework would be woefully incomplete if it did not account for time constraints. This chapter has shown how to incorporate a time constraint into our framework in an analogous fashion to the budget constraint. There are two main takeaway points from this chapter with implications for nutrition and health.

First, changes in the opportunity cost of time will affect the demand for food. A substantial literature shows that as the opportunity cost of time for FAH increases, the demand for FAH decreases, completely consistent with the law of demand and the figures given in this chapter. See Davis 2014 for a review.

Second, some individuals may not reach a nutrient recommendation due to money; for others, it may be time. Consequently, it should not be surprising that money-only policies, such as the Supplemental Nutrition Assistance Program, which provides monetary benefits for food among eligible, low-income Americans, may be of limited effectiveness if the main constraint is time. This could certainly be the case for individuals who are working more than one job or who work in a physically demanding profession; they may be exhausted at day's end and do not feel like doing the additional "work" in food planning and preparation at home. Even just the perception of time pressure can negatively affect food choices and health (e.g., Beshara et al. 2010;Welch et al. 2009). As Nobel Laureate Gary Becker has said (Becker 2008, p. 47), "[I]n the United States, the opportunity cost of time may be more important than the direct cost of goods." Indeed, recent research has found that time is much more important than money in reaching dietary recommendations (e.g., Davis and You 2010a, 2010b, 2011, 2013; Yang, Davis, and Muth 2015).

What are the options for improving diets and health? All of the analyses to this point have assumed that preferences are constant, but a central theme of this book is that choices are determined by the interaction of preferences and constraints. We have only been talking about changes in constraints. If you cannot reach a target by changing constraints, perhaps you can reach it by changing preferences, which is the main premise of most nutrition education programs. Indeed, there is some research showing that changing knowledge and hence preferences can affect the perceptions of time barriers such that they are less constraining (Mothersbaugh, Herrmann, and Warland 1993). So let the journey continue as we consider how changing preferences are incorporated into our framework in the next chapter.

Closing Conversation

JP: Much of what we have discussed tonight is very intuitive. I really like the concept of a full price that incorporates a money component and a time component. I can see how that is quite useful in analyzing many different scenarios. For example, in our literature there has been much discussion about "accessibility," which bundles time, convenience, location, and even price into one construct. The research shows that someone who lacks "access" to nutritious foods is less likely to eat well.

Margaret: Interesting. In economics, we would keep these effects separate and not try to bundle them because each of those variables will have a different and unique effect. By lumping them all together into one construct, you don't know which one is causing the change in "accessibility." For example, in one case accessibility may be changing due to a change in the price of food and in another case it may be changing due to a change in convenience. The policy recommendation implications will be very different, depending on what is causing the change.

JP: I agree. I think the economics approach simplifies how to view choices. In the nutrition field, there isn't even consensus on how to define and/or measure "accessibility."

7

Information and Preferences

Learning Objectives

What you will know by the end of this chapter:

- ¤ how information is incorporated into the economic framework;
- ¤ how information or educational campaigns can appear unsuccessful when in fact they have just been offset or moderated by other factors;
- ¤ how the economic framework helps in identifying what moderating factors may be counteracting the education or information campaign; and
- ¤ how information can affect the demand for foods and therefore nutrition and health.

Opening Conversation

JP: [texting Margaret at work]. Thx 4 enjoyable night. Honey want play date with Blanco Saturday at 3?

Margaret: Sister visiting. Can she come?

JP: Y

[At park on Saturday]

Margaret: This is my sister, Ann.

JP: Hello. Nice to meet you.

Ann: Likewise. I've heard a lot about you. Margaret says you're interested in economics.

JP: Yes, I am. In fact, Margaret, something is really bothering me about this economic framework you've been explaining. Everything seems to be explained by constraints, or what we call barriers, such as income, price, and time. But what if something happens that changes what people like, what you called "preferences"? For example, most nutrition education programs are not interested in changing income, prices, or time, but rather trying to educate people about how to eat healthier. Are you saying those programs will have no effect in the economic framework?

Margaret: No, not at all. Preferences can change, but it's not precise in the traditional or neoclassical economic approach. It can be useful in framing the discussion about informational campaigns, however. Uh oh, my sister is rolling her eyes!

Background Material

Each day, we are bombarded with all types of food and nutrition information. Until now we have assumed what economists call perfect information. *Perfect information* means the economic agent has complete knowledge of all relevant factors for his or her decision. So we have implicitly been assuming that consumers know their budget, the prices of goods, their available time, and the nutritional content or nutritional target they are trying to hit. Of course, consumers do *not* have perfect information, especially with respect to food and nutrition, so as information changes, purchasing decisions can also change. This chapter will present the neoclassical approach to incorporating information in the economic framework. Contrary to much professional and popular belief, the neoclassical framework does *not* assume preferences cannot change, but instead challenges the researcher to be vigilant in identifying the ultimate cause of the change rather than just defaulting to a vacuous "change in preference" argument to explain choices (Becker 1993; Stigler and Becker 1977).

Information broadly comes from three sources: (i) the private sector, (ii) the public sector, and (iii) social networks. The *private sector* includes all business entities, and they disseminate information mainly to increase sales and profits. Advertising is the most common form of private sector information. For example, in 2012, fast food restaurants spent about $4.6 billion on TV advertising (Harris et al. 2013). The *public sector* includes all government entities and more generally nonprofit organizations. In the context of this book, they disseminate information mainly to improve public health and nutrition. Many of the resources we described in Chapter 1, including the DGAs, MyPlate, and the Nutrition Facts Label are examples of public sector information, but there are others, such as the Expanded Food and Nutrition and Education Program (EFNEP) and the Supplemental Nutrition Assistance Program Education (SNAP-Ed). Finally, *social networks* include all personal and professional connections through various social connections (e.g., family, friends, colleagues, etc.) and entities (e.g. workplace, social organizations, etc.). Information dissemination may differ for each of these sources by medium (e.g., print, TV, billboard, online, face-to-face), purpose (e.g., educational, advocacy, promotional), and of course quality (e.g., accurate, inaccurate). Regardless of the source, medium, or type of information, the overall goal across these is ultimately the same: to provide information that may influence food purchases and consumption.

Across disciplines the general logic chain for how information affects choices is the same: *Information is disseminated* ⇒ *Information is consumed* ⇒ *Information is comprehended* ⇒ *Different knowledge* ⇒ *Different preferences*

⇒ *Different choices*. If any link in this chain is broken, choices are unlikely to be affected by the information. For example, in 2010 it was estimated that the daily exposure to television food advertisements by age categories were children (2–11 years) 13.4 ads per day, adolescents (12–17 years) 16.2 ads per day, and adults (18–49) 19.3 ads per day (Harris et al. 2010). Clearly a child, or even an adult, will not purchase all items associated with advertisements, though the information is "consumed." Alternatively, a person may read (consume) with great attention that whole grains are high in fiber, but if she does not comprehend the role fiber plays in digestive and overall health, that information is useless. Continuing along the chain, a person may completely comprehend the information but ignore it because the source is unreliable or goes counter to her cultural, religious, or belief systems. For example, a Latina may fully understand that whole-grain tortillas are more nutritious, but because she and her husband were raised with (white) flour tortillas, she may not feel comfortable switching.

The actual process from receiving information to changing behavior is certainly quite complicated and constitutes entire research programs within many disciplines (e.g., nutrition education and behavior, behavioral and cognitive science, psychology, sociology). Indeed, there are several competing and complementary theories of behavior change, such as Social Cognitive Theory, the Health Belief Model, the Theory of Planned Behavior, the Trans-theoretical Model (Stages of Change), and the Theory of Reasoned Action, that aim to explain health behavior change (Glanz, Rimer, and Viswanath 2008). Many of the factors overlap across theories, and behavior change is recognized as a process requiring multiple steps.

In contrast to these other disciplines, the neoclassical economics approach to information and behavior change is not too concerned with the actual process.[1] Why? Because the focus of the neoclassical economics approach is on the effect, the outcome, and the actual choices made, not necessarily how the individual got there. One does not have to understand a process to observe an effect. Perhaps a non-food analogy will help. Suppose you know nothing, and we mean *nothing*, about cars. Your friend tells you that if you press the accelerator, the speed of the car will increase. How would you determine if your friend is lying? You would simply press the accelerator and see what happens to the speedometer or just feel it. You don't need to understand the details of the combustion engine process to check if the statement is true. Now, suppose the car did not accelerate when the accelerator was pressed. Now knowing the combustion engine process would be

---

[1] Preference formation and information processing is one of the weaker links in neoclassical economic theory, which places more emphasis on constraints as explanations than preferences, though preferences are certainly recognized as important. The importance of understanding preference formation is one of the longest ongoing debates in the economics literature. Neoclassical economics usually takes preferences as given, whereas behavioral economics and psychology focus more on preference formation and changes to explain choices. We will discuss these distinctions and implications in more detail in the behavioral economics chapter (Chapter 9).

greatly beneficial for determining why it did not accelerate. These are two different questions: *Does* the car accelerate versus *How* does the car accelerate?[2]

Neoclassical economists do not ignore information; they just use a simple modeling approach of incorporating information through its effect on human capital (e.g., Stigler and Becker 1977). *Human capital* is a construct that refers to the stock of skills and knowledge an individual possesses that will affect consumption and production decisions. There are generally two types of human capital. *Specific human capital* refers to skills or knowledge that may be useful for a specific activity but will not affect a wide range of activities. *General human capital* refers to skills or knowledge that may be useful across a wide spectrum of activities.[3] For example, there are many people in the world who cannot read (a general human capital item), but they are exceptional cooks (a specific human capital). Information can be targeted at specific or general human capital enhancement. Food advertising and food labels are examples of information campaigns that are targeted at specific human capital enhancement: knowledge and skills about food and nutrition. General educational campaigns, like No Child Left Behind, target general human capital, such as reading or math literacy. Clearly, the accumulation of specific human capital *may* be inhibited by the lack of general human capital. So how is information via human capital incorporated into our economic framework?

Analytics of Informational Campaigns

In the human capital approach, the logic chain above is simplified:

Information is disseminated ⇒ *the consumption of the information input may change human capital* ⇒ *a change in human capital leads to a change in total utility* ⇒ *different choices.*

Though we could give the equations, the ultimate goal here is intuition, and the intuition is more easily communicated with the graphical language.[4] For clarity, assume there are two foods: one "healthy" (F_H) and one "unhealthy" (F_U). Each of these has a full price as in Chapter 6 $\Pi_H = P_H + w_H T_H$ and $\Pi_U = P_U + w_U T_U$. As before, P is the money price of the food, w the money value of time spent on the

---

[2] Philosopher of science Nancy Cartwright (1980), in her aptly titled article "The Truth Doesn't Explain Much," states it more generally this way: "Scientific theories must tell us both what is true in nature, and how we are to explain it. I shall argue these are entirely different functions and should be kept distinct."

[3] Human capital in health is obviously closely related to the concept of health literacy used in the health sciences.

[4] Here is a sketch of the math. The utility function now simply incorporates human capital variables K that are functions of information I: $U = U(F_1, F_2, I) = u(F_1, F_2, K(I))$. The first equality gives the "derived" or reduced form of the utility function. So the utility level (i.e., the indifference curve) will now be a function also of information. If one does not like the human capital approach, an alternative approach is to include "taste parameters" that depend on information, which leads to the exact same derived utility function (Basmann 1956).

food item, and T the amount of time per unit of food item consumed. Figure 7.1 shows the effect a nutrition information campaign may have on the utility level and hence choices. The original equilibrium with no nutrition information is given by point O. However, after participating in a nutrition education program, such as EFNEP, the indifference curve shifts to the northwest. The new optimal consumption point is N, with higher consumption of healthy foods and lower consumption of unhealthy foods.

Figure 7.1 is useful because it can explain how an effective information campaign may appear to be ineffective. Let's consider a simple example.

Suppose Brad is overweight. Brad likes fried chicken and frequently drives a couple of miles to the Chicken Coop—a local chicken restaurant. After attending a health fair and picking up a flier about strategies for weight loss, he decides to start eating more salad. For the first month he was doing very well. However, last week he was given added responsibilities at work and now must work an extra hour each day. Around the same time, a new Kentucky Fried Chicken (KFC) opened next to his office where he parks his car. How does this new scenario change Figure 7.1?

Figure 7.2 shows the countervailing forces. Suppose Brad is looking at meal choices over a month. The monthly maximum calorie level target line is derived in the same way as the recommended isonutrient line was derived in Chapter 4. Each meal of a food option ($F_H \equiv$ salad and $F_U \equiv$ KFC) will have a certain number of calories, so just add them.

$$C = c_H F_H + c_U F_U : \text{Calories from two foods equation,} \qquad (7.1)$$

As before, F_H and F_U are the quantities of the two foods and c_H and c_U the calories per meal of each food. For example, a three-piece regular meal combo from KFC has 1,040 calories (Kentucky Fried Chicken 2014), while a homemade chicken and cranberry salad for two servings has 580 calories (U.S. Department of Agriculture. Food and Nutrition Service 2014). So if each of these represents one meal

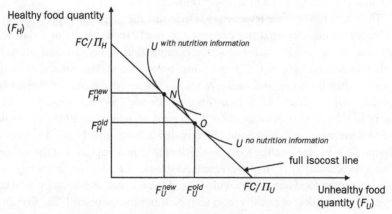

FIGURE 7.1 Full Isocost Line for Two Foods with New Information.
[IAPS] Nutrition information shifts the indifference curve toward healthier options.

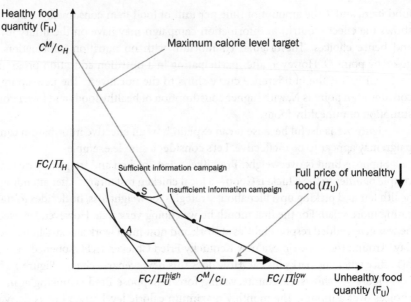

FIGURE 7.2 Sufficiency of Nutrition Information with a Decrease in Unhealthy Food Price for a Calorie Target.
[IAPS] The effects of a nutrition promotion campaign may be offset by a change in the full price of a food.

(i.e., $F_H = F_U = 1$), then the total calories from both meals is just $1{,}040 \times 1 + 580 \times 1 = 1{,}620$. Solving Equation 7.1 for F_H gives the *isocalorie line*—the tradeoff between the two foods for a given calorie level,

$$F_H = C / c_H - (c_U / c_H) F_U : \text{Isocalorie line} \qquad (7.2)$$

For every additional KFC meal Brad eats, he must eat 1.8 ($= 1040/580 = c_U/c_H$) fewer salads to hold the caloric intake constant. More simply, one KFC meal cost Brad about two salad meals in terms of calories.

The maximum calorie level target is then just the graphical representation of this isocalorie line. So what has happened in Brad's scenario? Prior to last week Brad was doing well by consuming the combination of healthy and unhealthy meals represented by point A and he was below the maximum calorie target. However, after last week, unhealthy foods (KFC) are now more convenient (i.e., T_U decreased). Furthermore, because his work life requires more time, his value of time in healthy food procurement (w_H) has gone up relative to time in unhealthy food procurement (w_U). This would be revealed in a statement like, "I can't afford to spend time getting healthy food now." All of this then implies that the full price of the unhealthy food Π_U has decreased. As drawn, the decrease in the full price of the unhealthy food has led to an increase in the amount of unhealthy food consumed *relative* to that of healthy food with consumption at point I. The maximum calorie target is now being exceeded for the given level of nutrition information.

The nutrition information is *insufficient* at point I to offset the reduction in the full price of unhealthy food. To get Brad to consume below his calorie target will require a more effective nutrition information program to overcome the reduced full price effect.

Alternatively, there may be some alternative program or the same program with a higher dosage that may lead to the new consumption at point S where Brad is consuming more healthy food relative to unhealthy food and still under the calorie threshold. Thus, at point S, the nutrition information program is *sufficient* to counteract the reduced full price of the unhealthy food. Note this graph demonstrates that a nutrition education program may work in isolation or *ceteris paribus*, but not in conjunction with other external factors.

What is the moral of this story? There are numerous factors that affect food choices. Just because Americans are eating less nutritious diets does *not* mean that nutrition information campaigns are not working. Rather, there are other likely environmental factors that are offsetting or moderating these positive effects.

A Pause for the Moderators

Okay, Figure 7.2 shows one type of moderating factor. Starting with Figure 7.1, assume that the new consumption bundle represented by point N is the recommended target. Can you show other changes in the full isocost line that would lead to *either* the same consumption level of healthy food *or* unhealthy food at point O? Can you tell a story with each? Here are some hints:

- What happens to Figure 7.1 if the *Full Cost* constraint increases?
- What happens to Figure 7.1 if the price of food at home (P_H) decreases?
- What happens to Figure 7.1 if the amount of time required preparing food at home (T_H) decreases?

Changes in the Demand Curve from Information Campaigns

Given that information can change consumption, as shown in Figure 7.2, then the demand for the food will be affected as well. So ultimately, the basic idea of an information campaign is to increase or decrease the demand for particular goods. Figure 7.3 gives a typical example of a demand curve for an unhealthy food decreasing as nutrition information increases, *ceteris paribus*. Of course, one could also draw a demand curve for a healthy food increasing with an increase in nutrition information. The attentive reader will recognize this as just another demand curve shifter similar to Chapter 6, so the mnemonic demand function device used there is easily extended to include nutrition information:

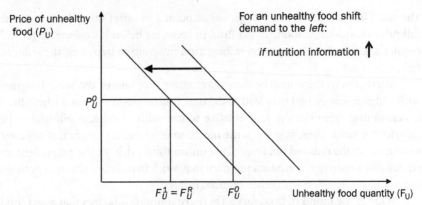

FIGURE 7.3 The Demand for a Food and a Nutrition Information Demand Shifter.
[IAPS] The demand for an unhealthy food is expected to decrease with an increase in nutrition information about the food, *ceteris paribus*.

$$F_1 = F_1(P_1 + w_1 T_1, P_2 + w_2 T_2, M, T, I_1, I_2)$$
$$\text{(-)} \quad \text{(-)(-)} \quad \text{(+)} \quad \text{(+)(+)} \quad \text{(+)} \quad \text{(+)} \quad \text{(+)(-)}$$

(7.3)

Demand function with information shifters

If you want, just ignore everything except I_1 and I_2, the last two variables in this math paragraph. Now recall from Chapter 6 that we had a sort of "all other factors" in the demand function represented by the variable ε. We are now simply being a little more explicit about some of these variables. Information 1 (I_1) is directly targeted at increasing the demand for Food 1 so has a positive relationship with the demand for Food 1 and would cause the demand curve for Food 1 to shift to the right, if information increased. Alternatively, Information 2 (I_2) is directly targeted at increasing the demand for Food 2, a substitute good, so has a negative relationship with the demand for Food 1. The demand curve for Food 1 would therefore decrease (shift to the left) if Information 2 (I_2) increased. Continuing the KFC example, F_1 could be demand for KFC meals and I_1 could be advertising by KFC, which is expected to increase demand for KFC meals. Alternatively, I_2 could be advertising for Chick-fil-A, which would be expected to decrease the demand for KFC meals. The general intuition should be clear: information can shift demand curves.

What is the magnitude of such a shift? Good question. Not surprisingly, that is captured by the information elasticity and will vary by type and dosage of information and type of food.

Conclusions and Empirical Applications

The intuition of nutrition information is rather straightforward. An increase in nutrition information should increase the demand for healthy foods and nutrients, thereby improving health. This idea is easily incorporated into the economic framework, resulting in the expected impacts on the demand for healthy and unhealthy foods and thus health.

Broadly speaking, empirical results support the idea that information affects food demand, nutrition, and health. However, the actual magnitudes, not surprisingly, vary along numerous dimensions (foods, nutrients, health measures, information type, medium, purpose, demographics, and analytical approach [i.e., observational vs. experimental approaches]). For example, advertising generally does increase demand for a product. The effect size, as measured by the advertising elasticity, tends to be rather small and inelastic, usually less than 0.5 (see Sethuraman, Tellis, and Briesch 2011 for a review). For food and beverage demand specifically, much research exists at the food group or product category level using secondary observational data to estimate advertising elasticities. Advertising elasticities at this level tend to be very small—often less than 0.05—and other factors, such as prices, income, household demographics, and general health information, appear to be more important (e.g., Kinnucan et al. 1997; Okrent and MacEwan 2014). One possible reason for these small effects is that observational data require a substitution of statistical methods for experimental control, and there is always the possibility the statistical approach is inadequate. Some recent advertising studies have taken an experimental approach and found a strong association between advertising and consumption of foods (e.g., Harris et al. 2009; Rickard et al. 2011; Rusmevichientong et al. 2014), and the advertising/health information effects appear larger than in observational studies.[5] Regardless, even if advertising's effects on individual foods are relatively small, one should not jump to the conclusion that advertising has no impact on nutrition or health. As we consume many foods, small changes across many foods can add up, especially if we consider the magnitude of individuals influenced by national advertising campaigns versus community-level information campaigns. Recent research shows that children who are exposed to more (unhealthy) food advertising tend to eat worse and weigh more (e.g., Andreyeva, Kelly, and Harris 2011; Chou, Rashad, and Grossman 2008; Gootman et al. 2006; Hastings et al. 2003; Lobstein and Dibb 2005; Mills, Tanner, and Adams 2013).

Broad-based policy-driven initiatives appear to show even less consistency than advertising campaigns. For example, in a systematic review of 31 studies on population adherence to and knowledge of U.S. nutrition guidelines since 1992, such as the Food Guide Pyramid, MyPyramid, and MyPlate, Haack and Byker (2014) found no association between knowledge and adherence to nutrition guidelines. Disparities in knowledge and adherence existed across demographic groups. Also, the presence of nutrition facts panels on packages does not appear to cause individuals to use the information; use has been found to vary greatly by socioeconomic and demographic factors (see Campos, Doxey, and Hammond 2011;

---

[5] The counterargument is that an experimental study may lack external validity (validity outside the experimental setting) and overestimate the effect. See the methodology appendix for an explanation of difference between internal and external validity.

Drichoutis, Lazaridis, and Nayga 2006; Hieke and Taylor 2012). Similarly, menu calorie labeling is intended to improve dietary intake in restaurants, but its effectiveness seems mixed. Some studies find a small positive effect (e.g., Bassett et al. 2007; Roberto et al. 2010) and others find no effect (Finkelstein et al. 2011; Holmes et al. 2013; Tandon et al. 2011). See Swartz, Braxton, and Viera (2011) for a selected review.

One possible general explanation for the lack of uniform results associated with broad policy-level nutrition initiatives is nutrition literacy. As discussed, information is one thing, but comprehension and implementation are two other factors. For example, related to the Nutrition Facts Label, one study (Rothman et al. 2006) found that while 89% of those involved in their study read food labels for nutrition information, the level of comprehension was much lower. Not surprisingly, higher nutrition literacy is related to higher dietary quality, and higher comprehension of food labels was significantly correlated with higher income, education, and literacy. More directly, Zoellner et al. (2012) found that a higher health literacy score is positively related to a higher Healthy Eating Index. Carbone and Zoellner (2012) give a good review of the challenges involved in nutrition and health literacy.

After reading this chapter, the mixed evidence for the effects of information on food intake and health should not be surprising and just underscores a central point of the chapter: an effective information campaign may be moderated or offset by some other environmental factor. In this chapter we demonstrated how a reduction in the price of an unhealthy food may moderate or even offset the effects of a health information campaign. However, other factors we have considered would have similar effects, such as time constraints, as found by Melby and Takeda (2014). Demonstrating and understanding the importance of moderators or environmental offsets should be useful for nutrition and health consultants who are trying to determine what factors or constraints are counteracting their message and what needs to be targeted in the message, as indicated by McCaffree (2001). So are there any more global concepts from economics that may be useful in developing information or education campaigns? Yes! Read on.

Closing Conversation

JP: You're right. The neoclassical economics approach to information processing and preference change is not very precise. However, it is precise enough to explain something I've long suspected. An education program may not appear to be very effective, but this may be due to other moderating or offsetting factors. This means that without the program, individuals might be making even unhealthier choices, correct?

Margaret: Yes. That is one of the appealing aspects of the economic framework. It separates out all of the effects conceptually and then reassembles them in order to determine the overall effect. The identification and separation of the different effects is extremely important when trying to determine which effect dominates and then what the appropriate policy response may be.

JP: Yeah, I can see that. And getting back to preferences, what would you like to do now? Go to my house for a cookout or go to a movie?

Margaret: Ann, what would you like to do?

Ann: If you promise not to talk about nutrition or economics, a cookout!

8

Now or Later

Learning Objectives

What you will know by the end of this chapter:

◻ what is an intertemporal choice problem;

◻ why food and nutrition choices are an intertemporal choice problem;

◻ why present consumption bias exists because of certain and uncertain delayed effects;

◻ some empirical findings regarding present consumption bias, food choices, and nutrition; and

◻ the implications of present consumption bias for nutrition interventions and policies.

Opening Conversation

JP: [on phone with Margaret]. I hope your sister, Ann, likes me, even though we weren't very good at including topics she was interested in talking about.

Margaret: She does like you. But remember, preferences can change!

JP: That's funny. When we were watching the fire in your fireplace last night I was tempted to ask you about the Marshmallow experiment. Do you know about it?

Margaret: Yeah. Isn't that from the work of the psychologist Walter Mishel, who gave kids the opportunity to eat one marshmallow now versus two sometime in the future? He found that the kids with longer wait times had better outcomes in many areas of life many years later.

JP: Exactly. I was just curious if your economics framework can handle issues of self-control and delayed gratification.

Margaret: Well, I think it is useful for understanding and exploring the tradeoffs involved. It is easier to explain with a graph.

JP: Of course, tradeoffs. Well, that sounds like a great excuse for us to get together again, but does it have to be a graph?

Margaret: Well, if it helps, it won't be a new graph. Let's meet at the park.

Cod Liver Oil or Potato Chips?

For centuries cod liver oil has been touted as having numerous health benefits, such as improving arthritis, cardiovascular health, and kidney disease, and even preventing rickets (from vitamin D deficiency). But cod liver oil tastes horrible. So an individual must decide if the bad taste today is worth the good health in the future. In economic terminology, there is a current cost (bad taste) but a delayed benefit (good health). Potato chips are the complete opposite: they taste good now but may contribute to poor health in the future.

When the benefits and costs of a choice occur at different points in time, this known as an *intertemporal choice problem* (*inter* = between; *temporal* = time). Intertemporal choice problems are ubiquitous in life (e.g., exercise, savings, college education, religious beliefs) and are studied across many disciplines under many different names, such as present consumption bias, delayed gratification, delay discounting, impatience, or even self-control problems.

This chapter covers the analytics of intertemporal food choice and its important implications for dietary quality and policy interventions. The intertemporal choice problem is relevant for food and nutrition choices for two distinct reasons. First, the normal health effects associated with a diet usually appear later, sometimes years later, such as in heart disease. So even if health effects are certain and known, there will be a delay. Second, there are numerous factors that affect health (e.g., nutrition, physical activity, environmental contaminants, genes, etc.), so the future health status associated with a specific food is usually uncertain. Both of these facts cause consumers to place more weight on the "now" hedonic utility received from food than the "later" health utility received from food. This in turn has important implications for diet quality and health policy.

Now with Later Certainty

Good news! The intuition of the intertemporal choice problem can be explained with the one food model you learned in Chapter 3. From Chapter 3, the total utility function was written as

$$U(F) \equiv h(F) + \beta H(F): \; Total\ Utility\ from\ the\ food. \tag{8.1}$$

As a reminder, the first part, $h(F)$, captures the hedonic component of utility, and the second part, $\beta H(F)$, captures the health component of utility associated with the food quantity F. Initially let's assume the health utility component and its value are known with certainty to the individual. The sum of the hedonic and health components defines the total utility function. In Chapter 3 we did not give any indication of the timing of these two utility components. However, given the discussion, the hedonic utility component, $h(F)$, provides utility "now" and the health utility, $\beta H(F)$, provides utility "later," even though the food decision is made now. The Greek letter β can then be considered the weight an individual places on future health in his or her total utility.[1] Because the parameter β plays such an important role, let's give it a name: the *delay weight*.

Note that as the delay weight, β, gets smaller, less weight is placed on the future health utility and implicitly more weight is placed on the present hedonic utility, resulting in a bias toward present consumption (i.e., *present consumption bias*). Figure 8.1 shows the implications the delay weight will have for consuming an unhealthy indulgent food, such as Krispy Kreme doughnuts.[2] From Chapter 3, we know that consumers will always consume between the optimal health amount and the optimal hedonic amount when they are maximizing total utility, *ceteris paribus*. That result applies here as well. The dark curve represents the total utility function, which includes both the hedonic and health components. The light curve represents hedonic utility.

To simplify the graph we have not shown the health utility curve. Why? We actually don't need it. The health utility is maximized at the recommended level of consumption F_U^R.[3] To maximize only hedonic utility, the consumer would consume the greater amount of F_U^h doughnuts yielding the hedonic utility level h^{max}. However, because the consumer is weighing both sources of utility in the total utility, we know that total utility will reach a maximum U^{max} between these two consumption levels at a point such as F_U^T. So, more doughnuts are consumed than recommended because of the pull of the hedonic utility, but not as many are consumed as hedonically desired because of the pull of the health component (i.e., health is given some weight via the delay weight β). However, note that as the delay

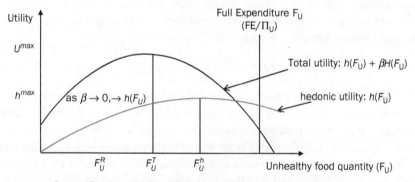

FIGURE 8.1 Present Consumption Bias Effect for an Unhealthy Indulgent Food.

[The IAPS] The less weight placed on the health effect of unhealthy indulgent foods, the smaller the difference between the total utility and the hedonic utility, and more of the unhealthy indulgent foods will be consumed.

---

[1] This is a very simple hyperbolic discounting model, similar to that found in O'Donoghue and Rabin (2006). There is a large literature on intertemporal choice and discounting in economics, with the seminal review article being Frederick, Loewenstein, and O'Donoghue (2002). See also Ruhm (2012).

[2] The terms "indulgent" and "unindulgent" should always be read as relative to some other available food.

[3] Figure 8.1 is a simplified version of Figure 3.8. If you would like to see the graph with the health utility curve, just refer to Figure 3.8. The text discussion here would apply to Figure 3.8 as well. In fact, this discussion is just the answer to Intellect Enhancing Inquiries #3 in Chapter 3.

weight β decreases, the total utility curve approaches the hedonic utility curve and consumption of doughnuts will increase, leading to greater overconsumption relative to the recommended level. Stated a little more succinctly: as $\beta \to 0$, then $h(F) + \beta H(F) \to h(F)$ and so $F_U^T \to F_U^h$. In fact, if the delay weight $\beta = 0$, the total utility curve and the hedonic utility curve are identical (see Equation 8.1). Finally, note in Figure 8.1 that the full expenditure constraint on the unhealthy food is not binding (i.e., the person has more than enough money and time to consume whatever amount he desires).

Now with Later Uncertainty

What does it mean for a food health effect to be certain? Well, it means, for example, that a consumer knows if she consumes an extra doughnut every day for a month, her body mass index will increase by some known amount, say 2%. Of course, not even a dietitian or medical doctor can predict this effect with this much certainty, yet alone a consumer. There are two general reasons why food health effects are uncertain. First, the precise biological process from food intake to health outcomes is not known. By "precise" we mean the effect is quantifiable and known with certainty (e.g., 10 additional grams of potato chips today will increase your blood pressure by 1.28% in 2 years for the rest of your life). Second, health is determined by many factors in addition to food, and some of these other factors will either accentuate the health effects of a poor diet (e.g., alcohol, smoking) or attenuate the health effects of a poor diet (e.g., exercise, genes).

Let's incorporate uncertainty in the analysis in a very simple manner by adding a *certainty weight* ρ to the total utility function:

$$U(F) \equiv h(F) + \beta\rho H(F) \ \textit{Total Utility from the food.} \qquad (8.2)$$

The certainty weight ρ lies between 0 and 1.[4] As the certainty weight increases, there is more confidence the health effect will be observed in the future. As it decreases, there is less confidence the health effect will be observed in the future. As the certainty weight decreases, more weight is placed on the hedonic utility and consumption is tilted toward maximizing hedonic utility. We again see a present consumption bias, but it is due to the uncertainty of the future health effect.

Figure 8.2 shows the implications the certainty weight will have for consuming a healthy but unsavory food, such as kale (in one person's view). The logic of Figure 8.2 is identical to that of Figure 8.1 except it is for a healthy food. The recommended intake and therefore health-maximizing amount is believed to be F_H^R, which is greater than the amount that would maximize hedonic utility alone, F_H^h, and greater than the amount that would maximize total utility, F_H^T. The individual consumes more of the food than he hedonically desires only because he believes

---

[4] For the mathematically inclined, the certainty weight ρ can be thought of as the probability of observing the health effect when there is positive consumption of the food item under consideration.

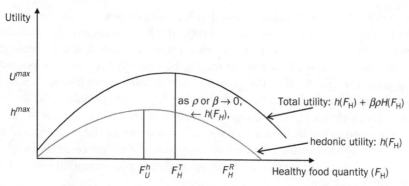

FIGURE 8.2 Uncertainty Effect for a Healthy Unsavory Food.
[The IAPS] The less certain the health effect for the healthy food, the less of the healthy food will be consumed.

it is good for his health in the future. However, as the likelihood of this future health state decreases, the value of the certainty weight ρ decreases, the consumer places less weight on the future health outcome, and consumption of the healthy food decreases. Stated more succinctly, as $\rho \to 0$, then $h(F) + \beta\rho H(F) \to h(F)$ and so $F_H^T \to F_H^h$. In fact, if the certainty weight $\rho = 0$, the total utility curve and the hedonic utility curve again are identical (see Equation 8.2). Consequently, this is consistent with a very general economic principle: people tend to underinvest in investment goods (e.g., health foods) in an uncertain environment.

Importantly, note that the implications for choice are similar for a small delay weight β or a small certainty weight ρ as both push consumption toward the hedonic maximum and show up as present consumption bias. Just observing a present consumption bias does not necessarily identify the cause of the bias.

The Healthy Versus Unhealthy Food Choice and Demand

How does all this affect the demand for a food? Great insight comes from just considering the "yes-or-no" decision between an unhealthy indulgent food, F_U, and a healthy unsavory food, F_H. Choosing a healthy food implies the individual believes he will receive more utility from the healthy food than the unhealthy food, or mathematically

$$U(F_H) > U(F_U)$$

(8.3)

Substituting Equation 8.2 into 8.3 and doing a little rearranging will yield

$$h(F_H) - h(F_U) + \beta\left[\rho_H H(F_H) - \rho_U H(F_U)\right] > 0$$

(8.4)

Consider the individual components of Equation 8.4. If the unhealthy food, F_U, tastes better than the healthy food, F_H, then $h(F_H) < h(F_U)$. So the difference between the first two terms—the hedonic difference—will be negative. But for the healthy food to be chosen, Equation 8.4 must be positive. So the term in brackets must be positive *and* large enough to offset the negative hedonic difference effect. This "*and*" part is extremely important. Again, it is not enough for the health effects of the healthy food to be positive; they must be positive *and* great enough to offset the negative hedonic difference. It is not enough to claim that a grilled chicken salad with low-fat dressing would be better for you at lunch than a big juicy burger. The health effect *differences* must be great enough to offset the hedonic effect *differences* in order for the chicken salad to be chosen. Note also that either a low delay weight β or low certainty weights ρ_H and ρ_U tend to reduce this last term, again pushing consumption toward the unhealthy food.

All the above analysis should be very intuitive and is based on the simple one-food model from Chapter 3. We could easily go to the two-food model looking at indifference curves, full isocost lines, recommended nutrient intake, calorie constraints, and so forth, but the ultimate interest lies in the demand for the food. The end result will be somewhat as expected. The demand for food will be affected by the degree of present consumption bias. Present consumption bias is another factor that would have originally fallen under the "residual factor" ε but now is explicitly recognized as entering the demand function and therefore the demand curve for a food. Figure 8.3 shows the effect of present consumption bias on the demand for a healthy unsavory food and the demand for an unhealthy indulgent food. As the present consumption bias increases, the demand for the healthy unsavory food decreases (panel A) while the demand for the unhealthy indulgent food is expected to increase (panel B), *ceteris paribus*. Remember, the present consumption bias may increase because either the delay effect or the certainty effect has decreased. In the next chapter we will discuss other possible reasons the present consumption bias may exist.

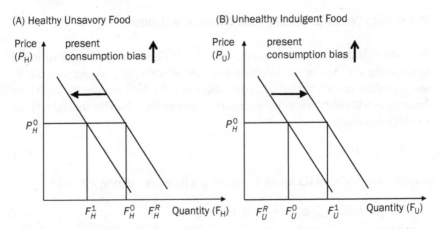

FIGURE 8.3 Effect of Present Consumption Bias on Demand for Healthy Unsavory and Unhealthy Indulgent Food.

[IAPS] As present consumption bias increases, the demand for healthy unsavory food decreases and the demand for unhealthy indulgent food increases.

Some Don't Delay Thought Exercises

1. Using Figure 8.1 or 8.2, assume the budget constraint is binding. Explain how increasing the food budget may or may not counteract a decrease in the delay weight or certainty weight.
2. Consider three types of nutrition/health interventions: (i) a worksite wellness program, (ii) a healthy food taste test, and (iii) a personal health risk appraisal checkup. Classify these according to which component in the utility function given by Equation 8.4 they target: hedonic utility, delay weight, certainty weight, or health production utility. Does the analysis of intertemporal choice help you determine why some may be more effective than others?
3. Using Figure 8.3, show how a tax on unhealthy indulgent food may offset or moderate a present consumption bias effect. In the presence of present consumption bias, discuss why a tax may be more effective than a nutrition education program.
4. Why might healthier AND tastier foods be an effective strategy for improving dietary quality and health with this framework? Explain.

Conclusions and Empirical Applications

In this chapter we have considered the intertemporal choice problem: making a choice now that has implications now and later. The two key elements in this decision are a preference for immediate reward (delay weight) and the uncertainty of the future health state (certainty weight). We demonstrated within the analytical framework that if either the delay weight or certainty weight decreased, then the food choice would likely be pushed away from healthy less savory food toward unhealthy more indulgent food, which in turn will likely lead to the negative health outcomes associated with unhealthy food, such as obesity. This points to the importance of offering good-tasting healthy foods to allow for both "now" and "later" effects to be optimized, without a tradeoff. So what do we know about the delay weight, the certainty weight, and their relationship to food choices and nutrition and health outcomes?

There is now over 50 years of evidence that shows that consumers place more weight on immediate (small) rewards over future (larger) rewards. This present consumption bias effect is robust in that it has been observed in a variety of settings, implying the delay weight is less than 1 and sometimes close to zero. In the context of food, nutrition, and health, recent research has shown that delay discounting (the delay weight) is important. In particular Rollins, Dearing, and Epstein (2010) found that a higher delay weight (i.e., the more weight placed on future rewards) moderated the effect of a more desirable food, just as would be indicated by our analysis. Appelhans et al. (2011) and Appelhans et al. (2012) found similar results for overweight and obese women. More work has been published looking at the relationship between delay discounting and obesity, and the general finding is that as the delay weight decreases (i.e., present consumption bias increases), obesity-related measures increase (e.g., Chabris et al. 2008; Dodd 2014; Weller et al. 2008). Epstein et al. (2014) found that a higher delay weight tends to moderate food insecurity.

As we discussed, the appearance of present consumption bias may be due to either a delay effect or an uncertainty effect. However, while a policy can do little to change the delay effect in the food–health relationship, policies designed to improve nutritional knowledge can reduce the uncertainty effect. Consequently, when designing effective policies it is important to determine which of these effects is most important. In recent work where both types of effects were controlled for, Andreoni and Sprenger (2012) found that present consumption bias was *not* due to intrinsic temptation or some other hedonic attribute, but rather the fact that subjects simply prefer present certainty over future uncertainty. In regard to nutrition, it is especially difficult to assign predictions for food and nutrition for later health benefits. Whereas some nutrients have "strong" evidence of links with disease, such as saturated fats and heart disease, other nutrients have less convincing evidence of health benefits for disease prevention or health promotion, such as the role of fruit and vegetables in preventing type 2 diabetes. Further, there are some nutrients with seemingly contradictory data, such as sodium/salt and total fat. Finally, referring back to Chapter 1, each food and beverage has different amounts of nutrients. So in sum, the complexity of nutrition as demonstrated in Chapter 1, a changing nutrient focus, and evolving evidence all tend to exacerbate the consumer's view that the nutrition–health connection is uncertain.

So, what can be done to address the present consumption bias? First, these findings highlight the importance of the science of nutrition, information dissemination, and especially nutrition literacy in helping to take the "un" out of "uncertain" related to health effects. Equation 8.2 provides a useful framework for discussion. One can consider approaches to address the issue directly by making healthy foods synonymous with tasty and indulgent, which amounts to increasing the hedonic utility, $h(F)$, from the healthy food. Of course, it must be the case that the full cost (money and time) of acquiring healthy foods and meals cannot be too high to exceed budget constraints. Programs and interventions can also be developed to reduce present consumption bias by increasing the delay weight, β. There is evidence that individuals can be trained to decrease their present consumption bias (e.g., Bickel et al. 2010; Mischel et al. 1989). Unfortunately, many nutrition education programs target solely the certainty weight, ρ, which would likely be less effective.

Alternatively, programs can be directed at costs, which are more immediate. One approach is to increase the cost of unhealthy food relative to healthy food, through money or time cost, to help moderate the effect of present consumption. An example of this is a "sin tax" on unhealthy foods (O'Donoghue and Rabin 2006). Another approach is to use a quality-adjusted price that incorporates the later health dimension in the price today, which is a certain immediate cost. Holmes et al (2013) found that expressing the price of a healthy meal in a quality-adjusted price on children's menus (a salient, immediate value indicator) was more effective in shifting purchasing patterns among families than simply providing nutrition information on menus (an implicit delayed benefit).

Finally, and a central point of this book, is that factors affecting demand often interact, either exacerbating or mitigating the effects of a single variable. This is indeed the case with other determinants of food demand. For example, Steinberg et al. (2009) found that adolescents, less than 16 years of age, discount the future more than older individuals, so the delay weight increases with age. Green et al. (1996) found that low-income individuals discount the future more than higher-income individuals, and this tends to offset an age effect. Coutermanche, Heutel, and McAlvanah (2015) found that as the level of impatience increases (delay weight decreases), body mass index increases and the responsiveness to declining food prices increases (i.e., demand becomes more elastic, so more food is consumed). All of this research suggest that individuals who are considered the most "at risk" and most targeted by nutrition education programs and interventions (young, with limited resources, and overweight) may have higher degrees of present consumption bias, requiring different strategies to change their eating behavior rather than just health information.

Given that the main goal of this book is to give you a framework for analyzing the economics of food and nutrition choices, you should pause to consider how this chapter differs from previous chapters. In Chapters 3 through 7, the factors affecting food and nutrition choices were mainly "resource constraint-based explanations of choices" (i.e., money, time, and information). The factors identified in this chapter describe the type of choice, not the available resources for the choice. The next chapter will continue to expand the list of factors beyond the standard resource-based factors that may affect food and nutrition choices by reviewing some of the main insights from the exciting field of behavioral economics. Let the journey continue.

Closing Conversation

JP: That "now versus later" framework is useful for understanding tradeoffs. It seems then that most traditional nutrition education programs are targeting the reduction of the uncertainty component of this framework. However, some newer programs seem to be targeting this present consumption bias problem in other ways. In fact, I've seen articles in nutrition journals citing "behavioral economics" as a growing field that seems to indicate individuals are influenced by many more salient factors than just income and prices.

Margaret: You are correct. Behavioral economics is a subfield of economics that is providing a lot of great insights on all types of choices. I have to get back to work, though. That will have to wait for another time.

JP: Wait. Are you just going to leave me hanging? When can I hear about this behavioral economics stuff?

Margaret: I don't want to wear out my welcome. I can't now, but I'll call you later.

9

Insights from Behavioral Economics

Learning Objectives

What you will know by the end of this chapter:

◻ the definition of behavioral economics;
◻ the eight main behavioral economic effects that influence food choices and nutrition; and
◻ some of the empirical evidence on the eight main behavioral economic effects that influence choices.

Opening Conversation

JP: [answering the phone]. Hello, Margaret! Well, after a week I was starting to wonder if I had done something wrong!

Margaret: No, not at all! I was just visiting my brother and his wife in Richmond. Last time we spoke you were interested in learning a little about behavioral economics. What are your questions?

JP: I'm in the middle of a project. Can we get together Friday night, say 7:00? I'll pick you up.

Margaret: Uh, this Friday at 7:00? I have another . . . Oh, never mind. Yes. That will be great. See you at 7:00.

What Is Behavioral Economics and Why We Need It

Have you ever wondered why most grocery stores have similar layouts and designs? Why is produce located at the front of the grocery store? Why is music usually playing? Why is there some enticing food aroma in the air, like chocolate chip cookies? The short answer is money. These are all techniques based on well-established behavioral tendencies designed to increase sales (Crouch 2014).

Behavioral economics is the field of economics that studies the interaction of choice environment attributes with individuals' psychological attributes or tendencies and the resulting choices they make. The neoclassical economics model discussed in Chapters 3 through 7 is silent on these environmental and psychological attributes and achieves most of its explanatory power by focusing on the effects of resource constraints (e.g., money, time, and information).[1] However, the field of behavioral economics has blossomed over the last 40 years and demonstrated that many environmental and psychological attributes can be just as important, if not more important, than standard resource constraint-based factors.

Behavioral economics lies at the intersection of economics and psychology and usually takes a more inductive approach to analyzing choices than neoclassical economics, which takes a more deductive approach. Inductive reasoning proceeds from first documenting specific instances and then drawing broader generalizations, whereas deductive reasoning proceeds from a broad generalization or theory to a specific application.[2] As a result, the behavioral economics literature is replete with a bewildering list of specific instances of "biases" or "effects."[3] We focus on eight effects that seem most relevant for poor food and nutrition choices.

There are two important caveats before proceeding. First, the effect definitions in behavioral economics are not precise and often overlap. One person's default effect is another person's framing effect. One person's framing effect is another person's cue effect. Though frustrating, the insights from behavioral economics are worth this frustration. We will define the terms based on how they are used in the present context. Second, the literature on behavioral economics is large and could easily constitute an entire book. The selected empirical examples are just samples of the concept in application; they are not intended to be comprehensive.

Eight Behavioral Economic Effects

A *behavioral effect* is a systematic and repeatable tendency toward a choice alternative resulting from the interaction of a choice environment attribute with a psychological attribute. The *choice environment attribute* is determined by answering

---

[1] Indeed, Becker (1962) demonstrates the law of demand (i.e., a downward-sloping demand curve) can be generated from just the budget constraint and random (irrational) choices.

[2] As John Neville Keynes (1917) observed long ago, scientific reasoning actually uses both inductive and deductive approaches consisting of three stages: (1) a first inductive stage where observations and data are gathered and then organized and categorized under more general causal headings; (2) a second deductive stage where general causal headings are woven into a more unified theoretical framework and hypotheses are deduced; and (3) a third inductive stage where hypotheses generated by the deductive theoretical framework are tested with specific cases.

[3] A search of the phrase "list of cognitive biases" yields numerous lists ranging from less than 10 to over 160 (Wikipedia). In behavioral economics, the terms "bias" and "effects" are used somewhat interchangeably. We prefer to use "effects" over "bias." "Bias" has a subjective connotation that leads down a thorny philosophical path about defining rationality that is impertinent for this text, not very constructive or progressive, and fortunately now somewhat dated.

questions: What choices are presented? How are the choices presented? What information about the choices is presented? How is the information about the choices presented? The *psychological attribute* is a psychologically based behavioral tendency triggered in alternative choice environments. For example, the present consumption bias effect in Chapter 8 can be considered a behavioral effect. The choice environment was an intertemporal choice. The psychological attribute was a tendency to prefer immediate rewards over delayed rewards and delayed costs over present costs (i.e., present consumption bias).

ENVIRONMENTAL CUE EFFECTS

Have you ever wondered why relaxing music is pervasive in food settings? Relaxing music prolongs the eating occasion so you eat more. Sound in general is one type of environmental cue. An *environmental cue effect* is a tendency to increase or decrease consumption in response to an environmental cue. An *environmental cue* is anything in the food environment that affects consumption. To understand what may be considered an environmental cue, we must first be clear on the definition of environment in this context. *Environment* is defined as the circumstances, objects, or conditions by which someone or something is surrounded. The "something" in this context is a food item and the key word here is "surrounded." The direct attributes of the food item (e.g., food color) are technically not part of the environment. As there are many attributes of the food environment, the environment can be organized along many dimensions and there is no single agreed-upon classification system. For example, one system is to distinguish between the eating environment and the food environment (Wansink 2004). The *eating environment* refers to the ambient factors that are associated with the eating of food but that are independent of food (e.g., atmospherics, effort of obtaining food, social interactions, distractions). In contrast, the *food environment* refers to factors that directly relate to the way food is provided or presented (e.g., its salience, structure, and package or portion size, and how it is served). At alternative useful classification scheme is by distance from the food item, with a continuum moving from the plate, to the table, to the room, the building, the neighborhood, the town, etc. (Sobal and Wansink 2007).[4] Regardless of the classification scheme, it should be recognized that environmental cue effects do not act independently but act in concert.

Most environmental cues are targeted at the senses (i.e., visual, auditory, olfactory, tactile, taste) and so the effects are often mediated through the senses. All of the following environmental cues tend to *increase* food consumption:

- convenience/proximity of food (Wadhera and Capaldi-Phillips 2014; Wansink, Painter, and Lee 2006);
- pleasant odor (e.g., Bragulat et al. 2010; Fedoroff, Polivy, and Herman 2003);

---

[4] Ambience effects (e.g., Stroebele and De Castro 2004) and contextual effects (e.g., Cohen and Babey 2012) would fall under this more general heading of environmental effects.

- larger portion size, serving dishes, and packages (e.g., Birch, Savage, and Fisher 2015; Rolls, Morris, and Roe 2002; Wansink and Kim 2005; Zlatevska, Dubelaar, and Holden 2014);
- background music or noise (e.g., Caldwell and Hibbert 2002; Woods et al. 2011);
- soft lighting (Scheibehenne, Todd and Wansink, 2010; Wadhera and Capaldi-Phillips 2014); and
- socialization (De Castro 1994; Herman and Polivy 2005).

While many of these effects may appear obvious, others are more inconspicuous. For example, larger utensil sizes (e.g., spoon) lead to larger portion sizes (e.g., Wansink, Ittersum, and Painter 2006); transparent packaging is associated with higher food consumption, especially for appealing foods (Deng and Srinivasan 2013); red plates tend to be associated with eating less (Bruno et al. 2013); and simply changing the clock to a meal time prematurely triggers additional consumption for obese individuals (Schachter and Gross 1968).

Environmental cues operate through three main channels: (1) they can trigger biological responses that affect appetite and hunger; (2) they serve as normative benchmarks for determining normal consumption; and (3) they can disrupt the monitoring of food intake. Consequently, *any* environmental cue that acts to induce hunger, enlarge the normative benchmark, and disrupt food intake monitoring will tend to increase food consumption. Perhaps not surprisingly, the magnitudes of the specific effects are moderated by individual traits. The literature on environmental cue effects is enormous and growing. Wansink (2006 and 2014) provides an extensive review and documents many of these effects.

DEFAULT EFFECT

Suppose every week you meet a friend for lunch at Cindy's, a fast food restaurant. You always order the #1 combo: a hamburger, an order of French fries, and a soft drink. You have just encountered a default option. By definition a "combo meal" groups together food items so there is an automatic or default choice for the components. Alternatively, suppose the default drink is water. Do you think you are more likely to drink water with the meal if water is the default option? In many cases people will just consume the default option, even if a preferred alternative is available. This is an example of the default effect.

In its most general form, the *default effect* is simply the tendency to accept the option made available, even when some apparently preferable alternative is available. The default effect is mainly associated with what options are *presented* and how the resulting choices are affected.[5] A default effect is always associated with a default option. The *default option* is the option that is emphasized over some other option. Of course, emphasis can range from strong to weak (Wisdom,

---

[5] The default effect may also be called the status quo or habit effect, though technically these are broader concepts.

Downs, and Loewenstein 2010). A *strong default* is one where the other choices (options) are not easily accessed by the consumer (e.g., offering only water as the side, and the consumer must ask for a soft drink). A *weak default* is one where the default option is emphasized but the other choices (options) are easily accessed by the consumer (e.g., the default being water but the cashier asking if a soft drink is desired).

Research has documented default effects in a variety of food settings. For example, Wisdom, Downs, and Loewenstein (2010) found that when the default menu in a fast food sandwich restaurant consisted of five "healthy" featured sandwiches, and the full menu was sealed in an envelope available to consumers (a strong default), the decrease in caloric intake was greater than when the full menu was simply listed on the other side of the healthy featured menu (a weaker default). Thorndike et al. (2012) found that simply placing healthier items at eye level (a relatively weak default) led to increased consumption of the healthier items (e.g., water over soft drinks). Similarly, Hanks et al. (2012) found that simply introducing a healthy food line (a strong default) in a school cafeteria setting increased total consumption of the healthier items in the school. Just and Wansink (2009) reported the results of several different lunchroom experiments designed to improve diet quality simply by changing defaults. One of particular interest is a situation where a vegetable is required, but some students are allowed to choose their own vegetable (a moderate default) and others have no choice but must take a required vegetable (a strong default). One may think the stronger default would always be more effective, but the researchers found there was a higher amount of food waste when the students were not given a choice—which upon further reflection could have been predicted. So the moral here is that changing defaults may work, but a single default type will not work in all situations. Effective defaults are likely to be dependent on food, setting, and population.

FRAMING EFFECT

Suppose before ordering your #1 combo you see a poster on the wall that says, "our burgers are now 75% lean." If you are health conscious that may sound pretty good. Alternatively, suppose the poster on the wall said "our hamburgers are now 25% fat." For most health-conscious people that will not sound as good, so they are more likely to buy the 75% lean burger over the 25% fat burger, though both of these statements are equivalent. This is an example of a framing effect.

In general, a *framing effect* is the tendency for choices to vary according to the context and the manner in which choices are presented. Framing effects usually operate through what and how the information about the options is presented. The fundamental characteristic of any frame is whether it is a positive frame or a negative frame. A *positive frame* emphasizes some positive trait of the choice (e.g., the shot will save 700 lives; this item provides over 75% of the daily calcium recommendation). A *negative frame* emphasizes some negative trait of the choice (e.g., the shot will still leave 300 dead; this item provides 25% less than the daily calcium recommendation).

In one of the earliest studies, Levin and Gaeth (1988) found that simply label-ing beef as 75% lean versus 25% fat led to a more favorable rating of the beef by consumers. In a similar vein, Wansink, Ittersum, and Painter (2005) found that individuals who consumed a "Succulent Italian Seafood Filet" rated it as more appealing than individuals who consumed the same dish but with the generic name "Seafood Filet."

As we have already discussed in Chapter 1, foods and nutrition have multiple dimensions and frames can be formed in any of the dimensions. Framing effects can be important, but like default effects, they will likely vary by product, indi-vidual product attributes, and individuals.

AMBIGUITY EFFECT

Suppose one week your friend tells you, "You should order the healthier #2 chicken combo instead of the #1 hamburger combo, because that will decrease your likeli-hood of heart disease." You ask, "How much will the likelihood decrease?" Your friend says, "I don't know the exact number." You order the #1 hamburger combo anyway. This is an example of the ambiguity effect. You prefer the certainty of the good taste of the hamburger to the ambiguous bad outcome associated with that choice. Certainty is preferred to the unknown.

The *ambiguity effect* is the tendency for individuals to choose options where the probability of a favorable outcome is known over an option where the prob-ability of the favorable outcome is unknown. The ambiguity effect is a form of uncertainty and therefore the logic of Chapter 8 applies here as well.[6] Most diet-related diseases are not only uncertain but are also ambiguous, meaning the precise probability of the negative health outcome associated with the diet is unknown. As discussed in Chapter 8, this is easily understood because of the numerous factors that can influence health (e.g., exercise, genetics, medication, environmental contaminants) and nutrition is multidimensional. The interaction of all these factors leads to ambiguous health effects associated with specific foods. As a result, the individual is confronted with a decision between the certainty of a tasty food that is ambiguously unhealthy (e.g., a meat lover's pizza) versus the cer-tainty of an untasty food that is ambiguously healthy (e.g., a veggie wrap). Because of the ambiguity of the health effect, the health component tends to be ignored. Consequently, food choices tend to be skewed toward foods that taste good but are unhealthy, *ceteris paribus*.

There is really no research looking at ambiguity effects of this type for spe-cific foods, but this would seem to be an important effect as most nutrition advice is technically ambiguous because precise health outcome probabilities associated with specific food items are not known. However, there is some related research

---

[6] There are two types of uncertainty: those that can be quantified and those that cannot. Chapter 8 focused on uncertainty that could be quantified with a certainty weight. Ambiguity relates to uncer-tainty that cannot be quantified with a simple probability or certainty weight.

from the medical and food safety fields. Using experimental designs that hold the probability of the risk of the outcome constant across an ambiguous and an unambiguous option, a significant preference for the unambiguous option has been found when choosing a risky medical treatment (e.g., Curley, Eraker, and Yates 1984) or being exposed to the risk of foodborne illness (Kivi and Shogren 2010).

CONFIRMATION EFFECT

Suppose now your friend tells you that the #1 hamburger combo is not a healthy choice because the hamburger is "high in fat." You counter with, "Well I read that high-protein diets, like the Paleolithic diet, are good for you no matter what the fat level, so I am getting the hamburger combo." This is an example of a confirmation effect.

The *confirmation effect* is the tendency to search for, interpret, and use information to confirm a preconception and defend a choice. The effect is ubiquitous and appears in many forms (Nickerson 1998). With respect to food, research suggests that individuals consuming more total fat, saturated fat, and cholesterol are less likely to search for information on these nutrients than those who consume less of these nutrients (Jordan, Lee, and Yen 2004). As another example, many people associate the term "unhealthy" with "tasty." Raghunathan, Naylor, and Hoyer (2006) find that simply referring to a food as "unhealthy" rather than "healthy" leads to a higher ranking of expected taste and also actual taste. As we look for and interpret information that supports our prior beliefs and desires, this can reinforce continual consumption of foods that are tasty but perhaps unhealthy.

ENDOWMENT/LOSS AVERSION EFFECT

Suppose you have ordered your #1 hamburger combo and are ready to take the first bite. Your friend interrupts, asking, "How much money would you would be willing to accept to *not* eat the hamburger?" You say, "$10.00." Your friend points out you only paid $4.80 for it. You respond that you place more value on giving up the hamburger than you do on purchasing it. This asymmetry in value is an example of an endowment effect. The *endowment effect* is assigning a greater value to something you own than you do to buying it. The endowment effect and indeed the default/status quo effect are often considered special cases of the *loss aversion effect*: losses relative to some reference state are larger than an equivalent gain to the same reference state (Tversky and Kahneman 1991). Consequently, because you want to avoid losses, you stick with your endowment or default/status quo option.

In the food area, Levin et al. (2002) considered a very simple experiment where subjects were randomly assigned to a "build up your pizza" group or a "scale down your pizza" group. In the "build up" group the subjects were asked to start with a basic $5 cheese pizza and could add additional toppings at $0.50 per topping until they arrived at their desired pizza. In the "scale down" group (the endowed group) the subjects started with a fully loaded pizza for $11 and were told they could remove items at a reduction in price of $0.50 per topping until they arrived at their desired pizza. On average, subjects in the "scale down" group spent $1.29 more than those in the "build up" group. This amounted to about three more toppings per pizza on average.

Endowment/loss aversion effects are one of the most robust findings in behavioral economics, but it should come as no surprise that the effects can vary by product type (e.g., Neumann and Böckenholt 2014). Of special importance for nutrition and health considerations is the fact that the endowment effect may be stronger for hedonic foods (foods that are unhealthy and taste good) than for utilitarian foods (healthy but less tasty foods). In an impressive experiment Cramer and Antonides (2011) randomly assigned a hedonic snack (either a Mars bar, potato chips, or a lollipop) and a utilitarian snack (either an apple or a package of raisins) to 554 students at 27 different secondary schools. Thus each student got two food items, such as a Mars bar and an apple or a Mars Bar and potato chips. When offered the opportunity to exchange their endowment for another snack, 54% wanted to keep their utilitarian food snack but 76% wanted to keep their hedonic food product. Of course, as always, one must be careful in drawing inferences outside of the experimental boundaries, as this was a study of children, who are known to like sweets.

DECISION FATIGUE EFFECT

Monitoring what you eat and how your diet matches the dietary recommendations takes a lot of mental energy. Chapter 1 demonstrated the complexity of understanding and keeping track of the different dimensions of nutrition recommendations. Should I eat this food or that food? How many calories are in a serving? How many servings should I eat? How many servings of fruits and vegetables have I already eaten today? Wansink and Sobal (2007) estimate that we make around 200 decisions a day just related to food. After a while this continual monitoring gets old and you start to suffer decision fatigue.

Decision fatigue effect is the tendency for the quality or consistency of decisions to erode as more decisions have to be made. In a food setting, Vohs and Heatherton (2000) conducted an experiment to test the decision fatigue effect. The experiment consisted of two phases. In the first phase, half of the subjects were placed in a room where there were tasty snacks on a table and the subjects were told they could help themselves to the snacks (a tempting, multiple-decisions environment). The other half of the subjects were placed in a similar room but told they could not eat the snacks as the snacks were part of another experiment (a non-tempting, no-decisions environment). In the second phase of the experiment, all subjects were taken to another room and told they were taking part in an ice cream taste test. As the experimenter left the room, the subjects were told they could eat as much ice cream as they wanted as there was plenty in the refrigerator. What do you think happened? The individuals facing the earlier tempting snack environment ate more ice cream than those not facing the tempting snack environment. The authors interpreted this result as a decision fatigue effect, where the tempting environment depleted self-regulating or self-monitoring resources, leading to less self-control.

In a similar manner, Bruyneel et al. (2006) considered the effect of previous decisions on subsequent decisions. In the first stage subjects were randomly assigned to a choice group and a non-choice group. The choice group was asked to choose as many single pieces of candy as they wanted from six different flavors of candy. The non-choice group was told what candy to select. In the next stage, subjects were given the opportunity to buy as much candy as they wanted of a highly appealing type of candy (a positive feature). Also in this group, the price of the appealing candy was set much higher than its retail price (a negative feature). The results indicated that the choice group purchased more of the appealing candy than the non-choice group even though it was more expensive. The more tempting positive attribute dominated the negative attribute. So as a person faces more decisions and temptations, the quality of subsequent choices declines. Obviously, in a food-rich environment with continual temptations and decisions to make, resisting hedonic food temptations can be tedious.

PROJECTION BIAS EFFECT

Suppose you have just finished eating your #1 hamburger combo and your friend bets you that next week you will not be able to order a healthy salad instead of your favorite #1 combo. The loser pays for both lunches next week. Feeling very full of hamburger and yourself, you take the bet, claiming it will be easy. The next week you are very hungry as you skipped breakfast. You walk in, smell the fries, see the picture of the juicy #1 hamburger combo, and start to order it when your friend reminds you of the bet. You pause and then succumb: "OK, you win. I am still getting the #1 combo. I'll buy your lunch." You have just fallen victim to the projection bias effect.

The *projection bias effect* is the tendency for people to under- or overestimate their own future behavior (Loewenstein, O'Donoghue, and Rabin 2003). People tend to overestimate their future abilities, such as willpower, and underestimate the effects of future stimulant factors, such as pleasant smells or sights. Of particular interest for food choices is the empathy gap. *The empathy gap* occurs when individuals inaccurately project their decisions in circumstances different from those currently being experienced. There are two main types. A *cold-hot empathy gap* is where an individual in an unaroused state (the cold state) inaccurately projects decisions in an aroused state (the hot state). For example, immediately following a midday Thanksgiving meal you are in a "cold state" and will likely underestimate how hungry you will be the following day or even later that night, when you will be in a "hot state" of hunger. A *hot-cold empathy gap* is where the individual in an aroused state (hot state) inaccurately projects decisions in an unaroused state (cold state). For example, right after you wake up, when you are in a fasting state you may overestimate how hungry you will be in a few hours, say at lunch.

Research has confirmed the projection bias effect and in particular the empathy gap. Read and van Leeuwen (1998) conducted an experiment where subjects placed an order for snacks a week in advance. Some of the subjects were hungry (H = hot state) and some were not hungry (C = cold state). They could order for the following week either a healthy snack (e.g., an apple) or an unhealthy snack (e.g., a candy bar). However, the next week, when the snack was delivered, they were allowed to change their choice. The experimental design was balanced such that the following week the snacks were delivered when some subjects were hungry (H) and some were not hungry (C). Support was found for both the cold-hot and hot-cold empathy gap. Regardless of the initial state, if they were hungry when the snack was delivered, they were more likely to consume an unhealthy snack. Alternatively, using observational data from a national survey, Mancino and Kinsey (2008) found that the more time that passes between meals, implying a higher hunger level, the more calories will be consumed and the lower the nutritional quality at the next meal. Similar to other behavioral effects, the magnitude of the projection bias effect will vary by product and individual characteristics. For example, Nijs et al. (2010) found that overweight/obese individuals pay much more attention to food-related stimuli than normal-weight individuals, particularly when they are food-deprived (i.e., in a hot state).

The projection bias effect is mediated by visceral factors, such as anger, hunger, thirst, moods, or physical pain (Loewenstein 1996). The most obvious visceral factors for food and nutrient intake are hunger and thirst. The homeostatic model of consumption is based on the energy balance equation and the signal to eat stops when the energy balance is restored. Unfortunately, this regulatory process is extremely complex and involves the interaction of external stimuli with internal sensory and metabolic processes (De Graaf and Kok 2010). For example, just the sight or smell of a food increases the level of dopamine in the brain and triggers a hunger state (e.g., Berridge et al. 2010; Volkow et al. 2002). Furthermore, our ability to monitor food intake is not very precise. For example, Wansink (2006) reported that a person can eat 15% to 20% more or less than normal and not even realize it. That is, individuals cannot distinguish the difference in intake over this "mindless range," so the projection bias may even be unconscious. So in a rich food environment where there are many environmental cues accentuating hunger and thirst responses, the projection bias effect tends to undermine good intentions of eating healthy.

Think Break

1. Think of a specific food you like to eat at a specific restaurant. Now give an example of an environmental cue effect, a default effect, and a framing effect that may cause you to eat more of that food.

2. Give an example of a food you eat where you suffer confirmation bias in continuing to eat that food. How can the information superhighway of the Internet influence confirmation bias? For example, what information can you find to support or dispute high-protein and/or high-fat diets? What is your confirmation bias story or argument?

3. On your busiest day of the week, do you make better or worse food choices? Discuss if you think this is related to decision fatigue. What

happens when you eat at an all-you-can-eat buffet? What happens when you are traveling away from home? What other settings might increase your decision fatigue?

4. Describe a time when you experienced projection bias.

Conclusions

This chapter reviewed eight of the main behavioral effects that are expected to be related to food choices: environmental cues, default, framing, ambiguity, confirmation, endowment, decision fatigue, and projection bias. These effects are manifested through an infinite number of mediums and domains, leading some to claim that in a choice environment "everything matters" (Thaler and Sunstein 2009, p. 3). This "everything matters" perspective is good news as it opens up a larger set of policy instruments that can be used to help improve the food and nutrition choices than are available with the neoclassical economics approach, which focuses mainly on resource constraints. However, the "everything matters" perspective is also bad news. A central theme coming out of the behavioral economics research is that choices are very context-dependent. This implies that economic policies will have to be customized to "local" conditions (environments and individuals). This is in contrast to more global resources targeted instruments, like a sugar-sweetened beverage tax or an income subsidy for low-income individuals. Finally, one can often come away with the impression that the behavioral economic effects identified here are at odds with the neoclassical effects found in Chapters 3 through 8, which is not the case. However, how the two approaches are related and if there is some broader analytical framework that subsumes both approaches is certainly not clear. While there is currently no agreement on a more general unifying framework, there are signposts from neuroeconomics pointing in a promising direction. Let us see where they lead us in the next chapter.

Closing Conversation

JP: Thanks for coming to dinner and for not bringing any graphs. Your overview of behavioral economics helps me understand behavioral nutrition interventions more. I must tell you, though, I'm now thoroughly confused.

Margaret: First, thanks for dinner. Speaking of environmental effects, the environment in this restaurant is very impressive—the candles, the white linen tablecloths, the soft jazz music, and the company. I certainly ate more than I normally would. Why are you confused?

JP: Well, for both being in the field of economics, neoclassical and behavioral economics seem so different. Neoclassical economics is very structured and logical. It is a rather unified theory, though I certainly can see limits in its ability to explain certain things, like plate size effects. The behavioral economics approach does not seem to have the same internal coherency and unity of the neoclassical approach. Is there a way to reconcile the two?

Margaret: JP, you are very insightful. There has been a lot of tension in the economics discipline over the last 40 years between neoclassical economists and behavioral economists. However, there are signs they are starting to realize the mutual benefits of working together.

JP: That is good to hear. Working together is usually better than working alone. Can you tell me some more about this?

Margaret: Can we continue the conversation as we walk down to Amore Café for some coffee?

10

Neuroeconomics

POINTING TOWARD A UNIFYING FRAMEWORK
FOR DECISION MAKING

Learning Objectives

What you will know by the end of this chapter:

* the unifying concepts for behavioral and neoclassical economics from neuroeconomics;
* the main components of the computational view of food choices;
* the differences and relationships between System 1 and System 2 processing;
* the influence of cognitive resources on choices;
* the importance of classifying stimuli based on the system that processes the stimuli;
* how a dual processing/dual objectives approach helps in explaining the different effects of different stimuli; and
* how the dual processing/dual objectives approach helps in designing and targeting more effective policy interventions to improve food choices and dietary intake.

Opening Conversation

JP: You seem cold. Take my coat.

Margaret: Thanks! That's much better.

JP: So what is the framework that unifies neoclassical and behavioral economics?

Margaret: Well, there is no completely unifying framework yet and there may never be. However, there are indications that the emerging field of neuroeconomics may provide some concepts that will certainly allow us to place the neoclassical and behavioral economic approaches under a broader decision-making umbrella. Here's how.

The Need for a Unifying Framework and the Computational Brain

After cataloging all the different behavioral economic effects in Chapter 9, one may resign to agree with Thaler and Sunstein (2009, p. 3) that "everything matters." But saying "everything matters" is not an explanation and is a vacuous theory. The most basic property of an explanation or theory is that it separates the world into relevant factors and irrelevant factors. The relevant factors are then organized under a unifying coherent framework to better explain phenomena.

The first generation of behavioral economists focused on identifying different behavioral effects and have been criticized for not providing any unifying framework (e.g., Fudenburg 2006; Gigerenzer and Gaissmaier 2011; Hayden and Ellis 2007; Levine 2012). However, viewed through a philosophy-of-science lens, the normal progression of science appears: identified phenomena are first classified, then synthesized, and finally integrated. Many authors now recognize that the most progressive and constructive way forward is to merge the strengths of both neoclassical and behavioral economics by focusing on commonalities rather than incessantly bickering about differences (e.g., Caplan 2003; Gigerenzer and Gaissmaier 2011; Loewenstein 1996; Rabin 2013a, 2013b).

At its core, an economic choice is just a decision problem. Over the last 50 years the computational theory of the brain has become a common way of organizing, analyzing, and understanding decision making (Edelman 2008). Simply stated, the brain is conceptualized as an information-processing machine that is goal (reward)-driven in answering decision problems.

All decision problems have four core elements: (1) the decision objective, (2) the information input (stimuli), (3) the information processing, and (4) the decision output. In a food choice context, the consumer's decision objective is to get as much satisfaction as possible from a combination of the hedonic and health utility associated with the food, given his or her constraints. The information input (or better "stimuli") for the decision problem includes all of the factors identified by neoclassical economics (e.g., budget, time, prices, and human capital-related information) and behavioral economics (e.g., environmental cues, default effects, framing effects).[1] The information processing is how the stimuli input are processed given the decision objective, and the decision output is the result or simply decision, based on the first three elements.

Clearly, how information is processed is the key element in this computational view of the brain because unless the information is processed, none of the other components really matters. *Neuroeconomics* is a relatively new field of economics that combines methods and theories from neuroscience, psychology, economics, and computer science to better understand the process of economic decision making and the resulting choices (Brocas and Carrillo 2008; Camerer, Loewenstein,

---

[1] We prefer the psychological term "stimuli" to "information" because "stimuli" is a broader term encompassing information variables, such as advertising, price, color, and so forth, but also includes things like plate size or music.

and Prelec 2005; Fehr and Rangel 2011; Glichmer and Rustichini 2004). We are in the early stages of these developments and no canonical model has arisen, but the cognitive resource allocation model is a useful conceptual device (e.g., Alonso, Brocas, and Carrillo 2014; Chabris et al. 2009; Kool and Botvinick 2014; Kurzban et al. 2013; Payne, Bettman, and Johnson 1993; Wang et al. 2010).

Cognitive Resources and Dual Systems

As we discussed in Chapter 9 under decision fatigue, making a decision requires effort or cognitive resources. A *cognitive resource allocation model* assumes that at any point in time cognitive resources are limited. Each individual attempts to allocate this resource efficiently across different decisions.[2] The current prominent view is there are two decision-processing systems (e.g., Kahneman 2011).[3] *System 1* uses a fast, reflexive, automatic, and perhaps "mindless" process that operates heuristically and expends little cognitive resources. *System 2* uses a slow, reflective, analytical, and deliberate process that expends many cognitive resources. While this modularity is conceptually useful, a continuum from 100% System 1 to 100% System 2 is probably more accurate. Some problems use mainly System 1 and other problems use mainly System 2, but often both will be used. In the context of this type of dual processing system, the cognitive resource allocation model yields three major implications.

1. COGNITIVE EFFORT IS MINIMIZED, IMPLYING A PREFERENCE FOR SYSTEM 1.

Given that System 1 uses fewer resources than System 2, it will be preferred over System 2 when cognition is effortful and cognitive resources are limited. After controlling for differences in benefits, Kool et al. (2010, 2014) presented evidence that decisions are made based on minimizing cognitive effort. For example, if the benefits of a specific decision are perceived as being worth a high cognitive load, then the individual may be willing to use the cognitive resources to make the decision (e.g., for high-value items, such as buying a home, buying a car, or booking an expensive flight).

2. RESOURCE DEPLETION CONTRIBUTES TO SYSTEM 1 USE.

As resources are depleted, individuals will try to conserve cognitive resources by switching more processing from System 2 to System 1 (e.g., Pocheptsova et al. 2009). This of course begs the question: What causes cognitive resources to be depleted? Cognitive resources are analogous to a muscle (Muraven and Baumeister 2000) and therefore become depleted with repetition and/or cognitive load (weight). Cognitive

---

[2] The brain claims about 2% of our body mass but accounts for about 20% of our energy consumption (Shulman et al. 2004).

[3] Dual-system models have been around for many years, go by many names, and can be found in several disciplines (e.g., Epstein 1990; Evans 1984; Strack and Deutsch 2004).

load is determined by how much attention, focus, and concentration a decision requires. Consequently, as decision fatigue sets in, System 1 is activated more frequently in an attempt to save resources while also making a decision. Furthermore, less important decisions will be relegated to System 1 to conserve cognitive resources.

3. HEDONIC DECISIONS ARE ASSOCIATED WITH SYSTEM 1, HEALTH DECISIONS WITH SYSTEM 2.

The type of decision problem can also determine whether System 1 or System 2 is employed. For example, if a person is hungry (a hot state), then an indulgent, great-smelling hedonic food will invoke System 1 because the hedonic effect is very clear and salient and the evaluation can be done quickly without much cognitive effort. Alternatively, an unappealing but healthy food that provides ambiguous health effects in the future must be evaluated using System 2 because the health effects are abstract, vague, and less salient and therefore will require more cognitive resources for a complete evaluation. Sullivan et al. (2015) found that the hedonic properties of food (e.g., tastiness) are processed faster than healthfulness properties. Given the bias toward using System 1, this cognitive processing bias then skews consumption toward the hedonic foods, especially when cognitive resources are low, which has been documented in several studies (e.g., Antonides and Cramer 2013; Shiv and Fedorikhin 1999).

Putting It All Together: An Integrated Schematic of the Food Choice Problem

So how does all this fit together to help unify the neoclassical and behavioral views on food choices? Figure 10.1 gives an integrated schematic of the different components of the food choice decision problem that is an expansion of recent work by Rangel (2013). Double-arrowed lines indicate two-way communications between the two components. Some stimuli will be processed by System 1 and some by System 2. System 1 stimuli are most likely those that trigger a hedonic sensory response and are quickly processed, such as stimuli targeted at sight, smell, or social setting. Consequently, we would expect the behavioral environmental cues, default options, and framing devices from Chapter 9 to operate mainly through System 1, because these stimuli are often processed quickly and sometimes even in a "mindless" fashion. Conversely, System 2 stimuli will be more abstract, requiring some type of analytical or executive function to determine the implication for the food choice. For example, all the neoclassical resource-constraint stimuli such as income, prices, and time would likely go to System 2 processing. However, as indicated above in the third implication, health effects require higher-level processing, so *any* other stimuli related to health effects would likely go into System 2 processing as well. Examples of these types of stimuli would be nutrition information (e.g., MyPlate, the Nutrition Facts Label, menu labeling) or statistical information on disease likelihood (e.g., the likelihood of heart disease).

Importantly, the two systems *are not independent* but interact, as indicated by the vertical arrows. A decision may initially be evaluated by System 2 but if

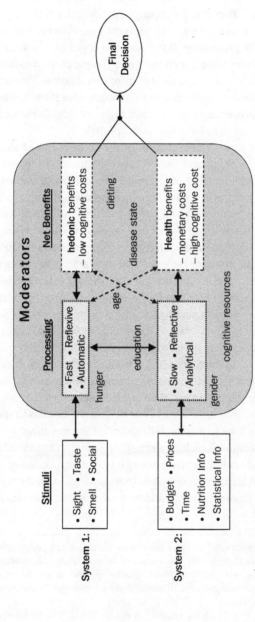

FIGURE 10.1 Dual Systems/Dual Objectives Schematic of Food Choices.

the problem is viewed as not worthy of much further processing, or the available information is inadequate, or as resources become depleted, it may be switched to System 1, effectively truncating a more thorough analytical evaluation. This provides a unifying cognitive process explanation for the default effect, ambiguity effect, confirmation effect, endowment effect, decision fatigue effect, and projection bias effect from Chapter 9. For example, the default effect, and more generally habits, can be seen as simply a way to conserve cognitive resources relative to the perceived benefits of processing. It is a waste of cognitive resources to reevaluate the same decision every time it is encountered if none of the decision variables has changed to a significant degree to be worthy of reevaluation. Similarly, accepting a default may be viewed as preferable to some alternative if the net benefits, taking into the cognitive processing costs, are not high enough. To the individual, sticking with a given choice may be *subjectively* optimal.[4]

It is important to recognize that all of the components of this diagram can interact in numerous ways, and the concepts of stimuli, mediators, moderators, and outcomes provide further structure in organizing these interactions.[5] In Figure 10.1 the stimuli are any environmental variables thought to influence food choices. These stimuli are processed by the two systems, which can be viewed as discrete mediating variables. The effects of stimuli variables will then be moderated (i.e., accentuated or attenuated) by other variables, such as cognitive resources, weight loss goals, education, or hunger. These moderating variables then affect the use of either System 1 and 2 but also will affect how much emphasis is placed on the hedonic versus health objectives in the decision making. For example, a higher cognitive load can accentuate advertising effects (Zimmerman and Shimoga 2014).

On a more general level, Mullainathan and Shafir (2013) reported numerous experimental results indicating that cognitive resources, what they call "bandwidth," are positively related to income: more income implies more bandwidth. Why? People with less money must devote more cognitive resources (pay closer attention) to spending decisions to avoid financial troubles than if they had more money. A single mother with four kids living below the poverty line has to spend a lot more time thinking about how to pay the bills and what she can afford for dinner than a single mother with four kids making $258,000 a year who can pay for a nanny, a personal shopper, and a cook. Effectively, the rich parent has purchased more cognitive resources by employing other individuals (outsourcing) to do the thinking in these domains of her life. Consequently, in addition to being limited in terms of how many

---

[4] The modifier "subjectively" indicates this is from the individual's perspective. This one modifier has significant implications for discussions and more importantly interpretations of choices and rationality. It implies the researcher should take a humble approach to research on choices as it indicates that what may seem suboptimal or irrational to the scientist may be completely rational to the individual making the decision.

[5] Conceptualizing and classifying variables as stimuli (predictors), mediators, and moderators is the business of science. The interactions of these variables can be quite complex and is beyond the scope of this book. See the methodology appendix for an introduction and Baron and Kenny (1986) for more extensive discussion. The central theme is that variables usually interact in determining final outcomes.

groceries can be bought, poverty also imposes a "cognitive tax" on poor people. So poverty pushes people toward using System 2 for only the most important decisions and using System 1 for what are viewed as less important decisions. Relative to other decisions (e.g., housing, utilities, or childcare), the immediate health implications of food choices may be viewed as having a low priority, whereas satisfying hunger would be more salient, consistent with Maslow's hierarchy of needs. Stated succinctly, ignoring the health component in choosing a food conserves cognitive resources that may be needed for more important decisions when income is limited.

Cognitive Effort as a Moderating Variable in the Stimuli–Demand Relationship

While Figure 10.1 is a very useful conceptual device for organizing concepts and seeing their relationships, it does *not* show what we can expect to happen to the demand for a food based on all these concepts. Can we translate these ideas into our earlier language that better communicates the more general principles? Yes. The main new idea is that individuals compare the benefits and costs, including cognitive processing costs, in making a decision. This is a generalization of the same fundamental idea underlying Chapters 3 through 8, so the translation should be possible.

Let's start very generally by letting $B(F_i)$ and $C(F_i)$ represent the benefits and costs associated with a food item i. The *net benefit* is then benefits less costs or

$$NB_i = B(F_i) - C(F_i): \ Net\ Benefits\ from\ Food\ i \tag{10.1}$$

Now, using the same argument used in Chapter 8, if the healthy food F_H is chosen, this implies the *net benefits* (including money, time, and now also cognitive processing costs) from the healthy food are viewed as greater than the net benefits from the unhealthy food F_U:

$$NB_H > NB_U \tag{10.2}$$

Substituting Equation 10.1 into 10.2 and rearranging yields

$$B_H - B_U > C_H - C_U \tag{10.3}$$

Equation 10.3 says that there are more perceived benefits in choosing the healthy food than there are costs in comparison to the unhealthy food. Proceeding in the same fashion as in Chapter 8, unpacking this reveals more insights.

Benefits are represented by the utility components of hedonic sensory utility $h(F_i)$ and health utility $\beta \rho H(F_i)$, so benefits are $B(F_i) = h(F_i) + \beta \rho H(F_i)$. The cost consists of the monetary cost (including time) $\pi_i F_i$ but now also a cognitive effort cost $e_i F_i$, where e_i is the cognitive effort cost per unit of food item chosen. For example, buying French fries in the grocery store deli may cost \$2.00 at the checkout counter, but they do not require any time in preparation before they can be eaten (time cost is low) *and* they do not require much cognitive effort, since you do not have to think about how to prepare them. Alternatively, a raw potato may cost only $0.05 for the equivalent volume of fries, but the time cost and cognitive cost are much higher.[6] So the complete cost is $C(F_i) = \pi_i F_i + e_i F_i$. Substitution into Equation 10.1 yields

$$NB_i = \left[h(F_i) + \beta \rho_i H(F_i) \right] - (\pi_i + e_i) F_i$$

Components of Net Benefits of Food i

(10.4)

Substituting Equation 10.4 into 10.2 will yield, similar to (10.3),

$$h(F_H) - h(F_U) + \beta \left[\rho_H H(F_H) - \rho_U H(F_U) \right] > (\pi_H + e_H) F_H - (\pi_U + e_U) F_U. \quad (10.5)$$

Do not be intimidated by Equation 10.5. If the healthy food is consumed, the *net* (perceived) benefits from consuming the healthy food, including the health benefits, must be greater than the *net* (perceived) benefits from consuming the unhealthy food. Let's start with the term on the right-hand side—the difference between the total cost of the healthy food (money, time, and cognitive costs) and the unhealthy food. Is this likely to be positive or negative? Given what we know, it is likely that in many cases the monetary *plus* time *plus* cognitive cost of the healthy food will be higher than that of the unhealthy food (e.g., the French fries example). So if the right-hand side is positive, the left-hand side must be an even greater positive value in order for the healthy food to be consumed. Is this likely? Probably not. We discussed this term thoroughly in Chapter 8. Humans are inherently drawn to indulgent foods that are high in fat, sugar, and/or salt, so the first two terms on the left side will sum to a negative number. This leaves the last term, the health effect difference $\beta \left[\rho_H H(F_H) - \rho_U H(F_U) \right]$. Given that evaluating health effects requires activating System 2 and there is an aversion to using System 2, there is an implicit aversion to even evaluating the term in brackets. All this implies that many choices will be skewed toward choosing hedonic foods over healthy foods.

To minimize your notational overload (are you suffering from cognitive overload and thinking about eating a hedonic food?), we have not written Equation 10.4 or 10.5 as depending on all the stimuli and moderators discussed throughout the book, but they *will* affect the net benefit calculations. And in fact, most of the stimuli that are mediated through the evaluation of Equation 10.5 will tend to skew choices toward unhealthy and indulgent foods rather than healthy and perhaps less tasty foods because of the preference for System 1 processing (i.e., mindless eating).

Let's cut to the chase: How does all this affect the demand for a food? The cognitive effort related to a food will moderate (accentuate or attenuate) the effects of the stimulus, depending on if the relative cognitive effort associated with the food increases or decreases. Figure 10.2 gives two examples. For Food

---

[6] Becker (1985) presents a model with time and effort as separate variables focusing on the labor supply decision. Effort is defined quite generally in his model, so it could include cognitive effort and indeed must in service-related jobs. The idea of cognitive or psychic costs is not new and goes back to Adam Smith (Chapter 10; Smith 1991).

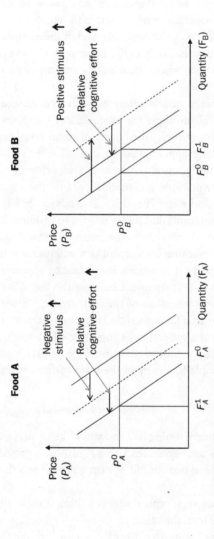

FIGURE 10.2 Examples of Cognitive Effort Moderating Stimulus Effects.

[IAPS] If the cognitive effort associated with a negative stimulus increases, the negative demand shift is accentuated (Food A). If the cognitive effort associated with a positive stimulus increases, the positive demand shift is attenuated (Food B).

A there is some negative stimulus that has decreased the demand to the dashed line (e.g., your favorite restaurant moved away to a busy downtown location with little parking), so the time cost has increased but the relative cognitive effort in choosing this food has also gone up (e.g., you will have to deal with the higher cognitive tax of dealing with finding a parking place). The increasing cognitive effort therefore reinforces the decrease in demand and the final demand is the solid line with consumption at F_A^1. For Food B there is some positive stimulus (e.g., a nutrition education program) that increases the demand for the food. But because the cognitive effort associated with the stimulus has also increased (e.g., calculating the calories in the food), the demand effect of the stimulus is attenuated and final consumption increases only to F_B^1. These are just two examples and there are two other general cases, where the stimulus and cognitive effort move in opposite directions.

The idea of a cognitive resource allocation model is a very useful construct for explaining some empirical findings. For example, for Chapters 3 through 8 we really had no explanation for why the effects of some variables we would think to be important actually appeared to have small effects on consumption (e.g., nutrition education programs, income, and price of substitutes). Cognitive effort provides *one* possible explanation because the cognitive effort effect can attenuate the demand effect (Food B). This obviously has important implications for designing programs and interventions to promote healthy eating. The behaviorally informed interventionist will understand that it is not enough to identify some intervention instrument that will increase the demand for healthy food, but it is equally, if not more, important to appreciate the cognitive effort associated with that instrument because the cognitive effort can completely offset the designed intention of the instrument. This is especially true, as indicated, for individuals facing a tight budget constraint. Fortunately the results are symmetrical, as a reduction of cognitive effort tends to increase the demand for a food, *ceteris paribus*, so reducing the cognitive load of healthy food is the underlying principle for many of the state-of-the-art interventions (e.g., Wansink 2014).

Some Neuron Noodles

1. Suppose you run a student dining hall and you'd like to increase the consumption of fruits and vegetables. Using Figure 10.1, provide two specific System 1 stimuli and two specific System 2 stimuli you think would achieve this objective.
2. In the context of Figure 10.1, explain why you think some of the stimuli may be more effective than the others.
3. Again in the context of Figure 10.1, identify two moderators that may undermine your objective.
4. Using a demand diagram similar to Figure 10.2, show what you think would happen to demand for fruits and vegetables based on increasing these stimuli.

Conclusions

The natural progression in science is from identification to classification to generalization through unification. Following recent advice, we draw on insights from neuroeconomics to present a framework that is broad enough to cover neoclassical and behavioral economics. Dual processing and dual objectives are key elements of this broader framework. System 1 is fast and automatic and requires little cognitive effort. System 2 is slow and analytical and requires much more cognitive effort. Food choices must negotiate both the hedonic and health objective. Normally, the hedonic component is evaluated through System 1 and the health component through System 2. The neoclassical economics approach is mainly designed to explain System 2-based behavior, whereas the behavioral economics approach is mainly designed to explain System 1-type behavior. The interactions of the stimuli, mediators, and moderators within these systems can subsume both behavioral and neoclassical effects.

So what are the implications for designing policies and interventions to improve food choices, diet, and health? As emphasized by behavioral economics, choices are always made within some contextual environment. The economics, nutrition, and health prevention literature is now recognizing the most effective practices, programs, and policies are those that go beyond altering some stimuli but also target the cognitive processing of those stimuli, mainly through the use of nudges (e.g., Guthrie, Mancino, and Lin 2015; Marteau, Hollands, and Fletcher 2012; Rothman, Sheeran, and Wood 2009; Sheeran, Gollwitzer, and Bargh 2013; Wansink 2014). A *nudge* is defined as any aspect of the choice architecture that alters people's behavior in a predictable way without forbidding any options or significantly changing their economic incentives (Thaler and Sunstein 2009, p. 6).[7] Common types of nudges are changing environmental cues (e.g., reduce plate size), default options (apple slices side rather than French fries), and framing effects (e.g., more evocative names for healthy foods). More generally, this recognition leads to two basic principles for architectural design in the choice environment: (1) target System 1-type stimuli, as these require fewer cognitive resources (e.g., Wansink 2014) and (2) if System 2-type interventions (an education program) are going to be implemented, some technique for reducing the corresponding higher cognitive load should be provided.

Behavioral economists usually focus on System 1-targeted policies recommending nudges that are rather situation-specific (e.g., using smaller plates, changing the default to apple slices, placing indulgent foods like candy out of reach). Neoclassical economists usually focus on System 2-targeted policies, recommending resource-based stimuli that are more universal (e.g., sugar-sweetened beverage taxes, fruit and vegetable subsidies). Generally speaking, behavioral economists tend to believe that if a factor is universal, it is not that important (e.g., price, income), whereas neoclassical economists tend to believe that if a factor is

---

[7] A closer consideration of the underlying philosophical foundations of nudges reveals a philosophical and logical quagmire, and the idea has been heavily debated (e.g., Lusk 2014; Mitchell 2005; Rizzo and Whitman 2009).

not universal (e.g., soothing music), it is not that important. Both of these lines of reasoning are wrong. As explained in the methodology appendix, an effect can be relevant without being universal (e.g., soothing music) and an effect can be universal without being very relevant (e.g., a small tax). Given that individuals use a combination of Systems 1 and 2, researchers and policymakers should probably follow suit and stop bickering about which approach is better and use a combination of neoclassical and behavioral economic approaches to understanding food and nutrition choices, as suggested by Loewenstein and Ubel (2010). Both approaches have strengths and weakness and neither approach has come close to cornering the market on truth. In the end, the implications for improving food and nutrition quality with interventions is not rocket science and is quite simple: *anything* that will make the healthy food eating experience more enjoyable (e.g., taste, smell, sight) and cost less, in its global sense (money, time, physical and cognitive effort), will help improve food and nutrition quality. The opposite applies to unhealthy food.

This section of the book has focused on the consumer's decision. However, the other side of the market of food producers and retailers is just as important, if not more so, in determining food choices. In the broader market context where most food is consumed, not just in a school lunchroom or an experimental lab, food producers and retailers are the choice architects. If we hope to identify effective policy instruments, we cannot ignore and must understand their objectives, constraints, and incentives. The next section of the book continues the journey and crosses the border into the land of food production and food retailing economics.

Closing Conversation

JP: Fascinating! I had read a little about this in a recent review article, but this helps. I find the idea of cognitive resources being a limited resource and having a cost as being very intuitive. I know personally that when I've had a hard day, even if I have time to make a fancy multicourse dinner, I'm often just too fried mentally to do it, so I may only make a sandwich with sliced apples. I've also worked with clients who say the same thing.

Margaret: I know exactly what you mean. I think it would be easier to cook with someone else.

JP: I can certainly see now why taking into account the cognitive resources involved with some type of nutrition intervention is a critical part of the design of the intervention. The framework is also useful for helping to identify different interventions that may operate either through System 1 or System 2.

Margaret: I do have to say that this evening was so easy and relaxing that I'm not sure if I used System 1 or system 2.

JP: I agree. I think we should cook together and we can test this more.

PART III

The Economics of Food Production

This section of the book covers the economics of food production. The first step in understanding the production side is to understand the main five sectors in our food system and how they are related. Chapter 11 gives an overview of these sectors—from the field to the fork. A deeper understanding of the food system is achieved by viewing a food system within the broader context of an economic system and then applying some of the principles from systems theory. Chapter 12 covers the basics of production, costs, revenues, and profits under the assumption that the firm (farm) is a price taker, meaning that its price per unit of output is fixed, which is very common in many situations. Within this framework we focus on the economics of choosing the level of output that will maximize profits. This analysis leads to the idea of the firm-level supply of a raw farm product, such as broccoli or cattle. Chapter 13 quickly extends these concepts to all firms beyond the farm gate, noting the connections between each sector and the sector before it, such as the farm sector. We then consider the case where the firm may be a price maker, meaning the firm can influence the price paid for its product, which is more common when we get closer to the retail level. We then use this framework to address the question: Are healthier foods more or less profitable than unhealthy foods? This leads to a discussion of market segmentation and the distribution of healthy and unhealthy foods in the food system. This chapter concludes with an analysis of calls for corporations to be more socially responsible by offering healthier foods and ways in which that may be achieved in a congruent fashion with maximizing profits.

In contrast to the voluminous empirical literature on healthy versus unhealthy food and nutrient consumption, there is a dearth of empirical literature on the production of healthy versus unhealthy foods and nutrients. Consequently, there are fewer empirical studies discussed in this section of the book. The economics of healthy versus unhealthy food production is an area where much work is needed.

11

An Overview of the Food System, Economic Systems, and Systems Theory

Learning Objectives

What you will know by the end of this chapter:

◘ the five main food sectors in the U.S. food system;
◘ the percentage each sector contributes to the U.S. food dollar;
◘ the six questions all economic systems must answer;
◘ the three main structural elements of any economic system; and
◘ the five principles from systems theory that are useful in analyzing a
food system.

Opening Conversation

JP [calling Margaret]: Hey, Margaret!

Margaret: I was just thinking about you. What's up?

JP: I just read this blistering article about how our poor nutrition in the U.S. is the fault of "Big Food" and our toxic food system. I must admit it sounded compelling, but it also sounded more emotional than analytical. I grew up in Wisconsin but honestly don't really know anything about food production. I know you grew up on a dairy farm and you have a B.S. and M.S. in agricultural economics, so I was hoping you could give me a short course.

Margaret: I'd be happy to! I definitely believe that economics can offer insights.

JP: Great! So over the last few months we have only talked about food choices from the consumer's perspective. But don't those choices also depend on what is available, such as what producers bring to the market? And how is that determined? Can economics provide insights that go beyond finger pointing and offer a framework for a constructive and creative dialogue?

Margaret: To understand the food system, it's important to know both sides of the market. Let's start by going over the main components of the food system and then seeing what insights the discipline of economics provides.

Mom, Where Do Frozen Pizzas Come From?

Suppose your precious, precocious 10-year-old niece asks you: "Where do frozen pizzas come from?" What would you say? The conversation might go like this:

YOU: Frozen pizza comes from the grocery store.

NIECE: Where does the grocery store get it?

YOU: From a food processor.

NIECE: What is a food processor?

YOU: A food processor is a company that makes food items like pizza.

NIECE: How do grocery stores get the pizza from the food processor?

YOU: They are delivered by truck, ship, train, or plane from the food processor.

NIECE: Where does the food processor get the ingredients: cheese? crust? sauce? pepperonis?

YOU: The food processor may either make the ingredients, like cheese, from farm products (milk) they bought from farmers, or they may buy the ingredients from other food processors that make these ingredients from farm products.

NIECE: How do the food processors get the farm products from farmers?

YOU: The farm products are delivered by truck, ship, train, or plane from farms.

NIECE: OK, I'm starting to see a pattern, but how do all these people or companies know *what to produce, how to produce it, how much to produce, where to produce it, when to produce it,* and *where to sell it*?

YOU: Those are great questions. Ask your mom; my mouth is full of pizza.

This conversation reveals two general features of all foods that are ready for consumption. First, there are usually many interrelated stages involved in "producing" a food. Even if you have a garden in your back yard, you still must "process" the food by harvesting it and preparing it for consumption. The number and complexity of the stages in general increases with the degree of processing. Second, all food production, including your garden, requires answering six basic questions: What to produce? How to produce it? How much to produce? Where to produce it? When to produce it? Where to sell it?

Currently, there are rather heated ongoing debates about the U.S. food system and its impact on health (e.g., Bachus and Otten 2015; Desrochers and Shimizu 2012; Freedhoff 2014; Lusk 2013; Moss 2014; Pollan 2006; Story, Hamm, and Wallinga 2009; Stuckler and Nestle 2012; Yach 2014). To help advance these discussions, this chapter will first give an overview of the five main sectors of food production in a developed economy, such as the United States. These sectors identify and define the food system. As the answers to these six basic questions are greatly affected by monetary considerations, it is enlightening to see how much each sector contributes to the typical dollar spent on food in the United States. We then place the food system discussion in the broader context of an economic system and systems theory, similar in spirit to Sobal, Khan, and Bisogni (1998). Placing the discussion in this broader context helps promote a more constructive dialogue among different groups. The unifying principles from systems theory provide fundamental insights for understanding the production side of the food equation (see Chapters 12 and 13).

The Five Main Sectors in Food Production

There are five main sectors involved in going from "the field to the fork": farming and fishing; farm raw product wholesalers; food and beverage manufacturing; food wholesalers; and food stores and services.

FARMING AND FISHING

A *farm* is any place from which $1,000 or more of crops or livestock are sold or normally would be sold during the year under consideration (O'Donoghue et al. 2009). This broad classification covers every type of crop from vegetables (e.g., carrots) to fruits (e.g., apples) to grains and cereals (e.g., wheat) to oilseeds (e.g., soybeans) and every type of livestock from chickens to dairy cows to hogs. Because this definition is based simply on sales, it includes farms, ranches, dairies, greenhouses, nurseries, orchards, or hatcheries and may be a single tract of land or a number of separate tracts that may be held under different tenures. This is a very liberal definition of farming because $1,000 worth of sales is a very small amount in terms of farming operations. For example, if you raise and sell *one* feeder steer, this will make you a farmer, assuming a typical weight and price for a feeder steer (e.g., about 750 lbs @ $2.00 per lb). Given this liberal definition, it is no surprise that farms can range in size from a couple of acres to several thousand acres. The King Ranch in Texas is 825,000 acres.

In 2011, there were about 2.2 million farms in the United States, with sales of about $420 billion (U.S. Department of Agriculture, National Agricultural Statistics Service 2011). Farm products are often referred to as raw products in the food industry and would be the source of the raw products used in the pizza example (e.g., milk for cheese, wheat for the crust, tomatoes and sugar cane for the sauce).

The *fishing* sector is defined as establishments primarily engaged in the commercial catching or taking of finfish, shellfish, or miscellaneous marine products from a natural habitat, such as bluefish, eels, salmon, tuna, clams, crabs, lobsters, mussels, oysters, shrimp, frogs, sea urchins, and turtles (U.S. Census Bureau, North American Industry Classification System [NAICS] 2012). In 2007, there were about 68,000 fishing enterprises in the United States, with annual sales around $5 billion (U.S. Census Bureau 2007).[1]

FARM RAW PRODUCT WHOLESALERS

A *wholesaler* is one who sells goods to someone other than the final consumer. The primary function of a wholesaler is the distribution and logistics involved in moving goods from one source to another. *Farm raw product wholesalers* are establishments primarily engaged in the distribution of agricultural products (except raw milk, live poultry, and fresh fruit and vegetables), such as grains, field beans, livestock, and other farm product raw materials, excluding seeds (U.S. Census Bureau, NAICS 2012). In 2007 there were about 8,000 enterprises in this sector with sales of $168 billion (U.S. Census Bureau 2007). Many firms that fall within this category are small independent operators.

FOOD AND BEVERAGE MANUFACTURING

Manufacturing is the making of goods using some combination of materials, labor, energy, and machinery, especially on a large scale. Enterprises in the *food and beverage manufacturing sector* transform livestock and agricultural products into products for intermediate or final consumption. Food manufacturing is often called food processing. The food products manufactured in these establishments are typically sold to wholesalers or retailers for distribution to consumers. Beverage manufacturing includes (1) those that manufacture nonalcoholic beverages, (2) those that manufacture alcoholic beverages through the fermentation process, and (3) those that produce distilled alcoholic beverages (U.S. Census Bureau, NAICS 2012). In 2007 there were about 55,000 enterprises in these two sectors, with sales of $675 billion (U.S. Census Bureau 2007). Examples of food and beverage manufacturers would be General Mills, Kraft Foods, Nestlé, Smithfield, Tyson Foods, Anheuser-Busch, Coca-Cola, and PepsiCo. Often these larger manufacturers will own smaller food and beverage companies that offer a variety of products and brands. For example, the Nestlé Corporation makes the home frozen pizza brand known as DiGiorno.

FOOD WHOLESALING

Food wholesaling is the component of food marketing where goods are assembled, stored, and transported to customers, including retailers, food service operators, other wholesalers, government, and other types of businesses (U.S. Department of Agriculture, Economic Research Service 2014f). Food wholesaling serves the two main types of retail food outlets: food and beverage stores (e.g., grocery stores)

---

[1] Many of the numbers given in this chapter come from the U.S. Census Bureau's Survey of Business Owners 2007. At the time of the writing they were the most recent data available.

and food services (e.g., restaurants).[2] In 2007 food wholesaling consisted of about 56,000 enterprises with sales of $672 billion (U.S. Census Bureau 2007).

FOOD RETAILING

Food retailing is the selling of foods and beverages directly to consumers. There are two general categories of food retailers: food stores and food services. *Food (and beverage) stores* sell food and beverage products from fixed point-of-sale locations. Establishments in this subsector have special equipment (e.g., freezers, refrigerated display cases, refrigerators) for displaying food and beverage goods. Grocery stores, supermarkets, convenience stores, produce markets, meat markets, retail bakeries, and specialty food stores, such as candy stores, all fall into this category. Beverage stores are primarily engaged in packaged alcoholic beverages, such as ale, beer, wine, and liquor (U.S. Census Bureau, NAICS 2012). *Food services* establishments prepare meals, snacks, and beverages to customer order for immediate on-premises and off-premises consumption (U.S. Census Bureau, NAICS 2012) and thus would include full-service restaurants, coffee shops, bakeries, fast food outlets, caterers, and other places that prepare, serve, and sell food to the general public. This would also include hotels, motels, amusement parks, movie theatres, casinos, and so forth. In 2007 food retailing consisted of about 890,000 enterprises with sales of $1 trillion (U.S. Census Bureau 2007).

Figure 11.1 gives a schematic of the five main food sectors involved in going from farm to fork. It depicts the food system or what is also called the supply chain. The dollar amounts in Figure 11.1 are sales or revenue, not profits. We will explain the importance of this distinction in great detail in Chapters 12 and 13. The key point of the diagram is the flow and transformation of goods from raw products to final food items. Importantly, this general flow structure will apply at all spatial levels, from the home garden, to the local farmers' market, to regional, domestic, or international food markets, with some stages being more or less important depending on the specific market (e.g., your 10-year-old niece may be the "raw product wholesaler" who brings in the carrots from the garden).

If a sector is observed in a specific market, then it is providing some service that is valued within the market; otherwise it would not exist. So how much does each sector contribute to the entire system?

The Food Dollar

The value each sector contributes to the system is measured by the food dollar and industry group series. The U.S. Department of Agriculture's *food dollar series*

---

[2] Most of this food wholesaling section comes from the USDA Economic Research Service website. There are several subclassifications of food wholesaling, depending on the type of business they serve and the type of products they sell. For our discussion these subclassifications are not needed, but they can be found at the USDA website.

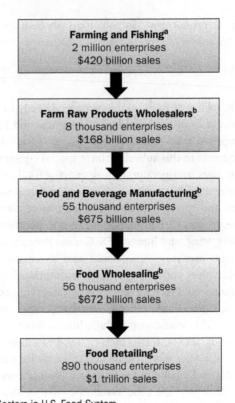

FIGURE 11.1 Major Sectors in U.S. Food System.

Source: [a]U.S. Department of Agriculture Statistics 2011. [b]U.S. Census Bureau 2007.[a,b]Author's calculations.

measures annual expenditures by U.S. consumers on domestically produced foods (U.S. Department of Agriculture, Economic Research Service, Food Dollar Series 2015). The *industry group series* gives the contribution to the food dollar—the value added—from 10 distinct food supply chain industry groups (Canning 2011): farm and agribusiness, food processing, food retailing (e.g., grocery stores), food services (e.g., restaurants), transportation, energy, packing, finance and insurance, advertising, and legal, accounting, and bookkeeping. Note that the transportation, energy, packing, finance and insurance, advertising, and legal, accounting, and bookkeeping sectors contribute to other sectors of the economy as well, not just the food sector. Consequently, these 10 industry groups do *not* match exactly the five sectors given in Figure 11.1, but the overlap is sufficient to demonstrate the contribution each sector makes to the food dollar.

As was discussed in Chapter 6, food consumption expenditures in the United States are now almost evenly split between food at home (FAH) and food away from home (FAFH), so it is useful to look at the food dollar decomposition in these two markets separately. Figure 11.2 gives the industry group value-added decomposition for FAFH in 2012 in the United States. Because the food dollar series is expressed in cents and a dollar is 100 cents, the numbers can be interpreted as percentages.

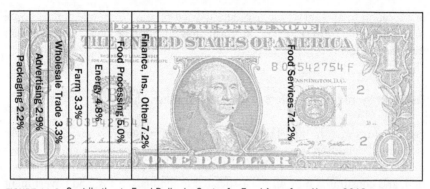

FIGURE 11.2 Contribution to Food Dollar by Sector for Food Away from Home, 2012.

Source: Industry Series. US Department of Agriculture, Economic Research Service, Food Dollar Series (2015) and author's calculations.

Ponder these numbers for a moment. Farm production provides the actual raw food inputs (e.g., tomatoes, milk for cheese, wheat for crust), but only 3.3% of the value of FAFH is associated with the food input. The other 96.7% is associated with non-food inputs, such as packaging for tomatoes, milling of wheat, transportation of products, labor in assembling the frozen pizza, and so forth. Are food services actually selling food or something else?

Figure 11.3 gives the industry group value-added decomposition for FAH in 2012 in the United States. FAH is food coming mainly from food stores (e.g., grocery stores), which requires much more at-home "assembly" via preparation and cooking. Not surprisingly, the value associated with the actual food (18.2%) is higher in the FAH market than in the FAFH market. But still, 81.8% of the dollar value of FAH is associated with non-food inputs. Again, we must ask: What are we really buying when we go to the grocery store, food or something else?

The answer is marketing services. *Food marketing services* are *any* food services that exist between the farmer and the final consumer. Marketing services can be broken down along three general lines: space (e.g., simple transportation from

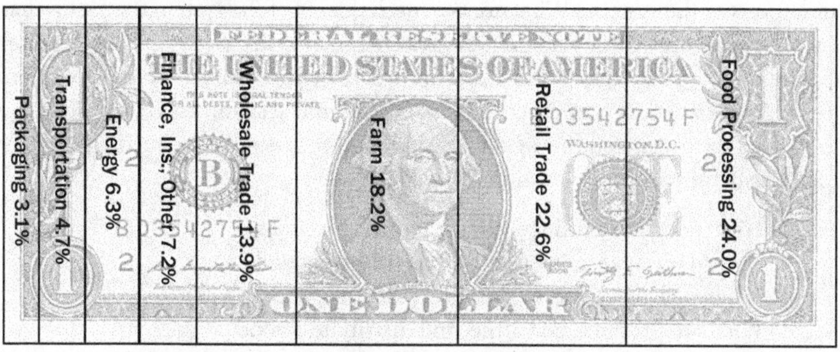

FIGURE 11.3 Contribution to Food Dollar by Sector for Food at Home, 2012.

Source: Industry Series, U.S. Department of Agriculture, Economic Research Service, Food Dollar Series (2015) and author's calculations.

one location to another), time (e.g., storage of a product from one point in time to another), and form (e.g., the transformation of a food or foods from one form into another form).

The Food System, Economic Systems, and Systems Theory

From Figures 11.1 through 11.3, the idea of a food system starts to emerge. Here is a formal definition. The *food system* consists of the operations and processes involved in transforming raw materials into food through production, distribution, and consumption by all the associated individuals, firms, and government agencies. As mentioned, the food system is also referred to as the *food supply chain*. The focus of this definition is on the operations and processes, not the entities, the location, or the scale. A food system may therefore consist of one individual on a deserted island, such as Robinson Crusoe, who raises goats for milk and meat. Alternatively, a food system may consist of a family garden, a "local" food system with a farmers' market, a regional food system involving a cooperative of producers and buyers, or a global food system involving the importing and exporting of products from one country to the other. Consequently, because of the ability to produce and buy different products in different places, these individually identifiable foods system "streams" or subsystems will intersect, creating the more general food system that incorporates these individual subsystems or streams. For example, most local grocery stores are part of a global food system that supplies food from all over the world (e.g., strawberries from Florida in January), but the local grocery store may actually be supplied with products from both the local farmers and a global wholesaler. Thus the task of defining the food system that serves a certain location or provides a specific product will often have vague boundaries, depending on what competition is also considered when defining the system.

The above food system definition is a useful organizational and descriptive concept, but it does not explain why and how the system operates. Why does the system exist in its current form? What are the benefits of the system? What are the limitations of the system? What are the mechanisms of the system that act as barriers or opportunities for changing the system? Answering these types of questions requires placing a food system within the broader context of an economic system.

A food system is a microcosm of an economic system. An *economic system* consists of the organizational arrangements and processes through which a society answers six fundamental questions (Conklin 1991):

1. *What* goods to produce, consume, and distribute
2. *How* to produce, consume, and distribute a good
3. *How much* of a good to produce, consume, and distribute
4. *Where* to produce, consume, and distribute a good
5. *When* to produce, consume, and distribute a good
6. *For whom* to produce, consume, and distribute a good

Each of these six questions must be answered at each stage in the food system. A gardening family in New Jersey, a corn farmer in Iowa, a global food processor in Geneva, a local grocery store in Ohio, or a chain restaurant in Texas must each answer all of these questions. But *how* do they answer these questions?

Suppose you are a member of a family of four and you are considering growing a garden. What is the process you go through to answer these questions? Before you arrive at these questions, you would probably first identify some motivation for wanting to grow a garden. Perhaps you enjoy working with the soil or you just want to eat fresh vegetables this summer. You and the family have some objective or objectives. But given there are three other members in the family, you also need to decide on the decision-making process: Dad the dictator? Mom the monarch? Or is it some democratic process? Finally, if your family has never grown a garden, you probably realize you need to do a little research, so you need some information.

This simple gardening example reveals *three core structural elements of economic systems* that are always present when answering the six fundamental questions (e.g., Neuberger and Duffy 1976):

(1) *The Motivation Structure*—the objectives for engaging in the activity and the incentives for pursuing the activity

(2) *The Decision-Making Structure*—the established arrangement whereby economic decision-making authority is allocated among the members of the system

(3) *The Information Structure*—the established mechanisms and channels for the collection, transmission, processing, storage, retrieval, and analysis of information required for making decisions within the system. This would include information on resource constraints.

Recognize that all economic decisions rest on these structural foundations. These elements apply not only to producers but also consumers. An efficient operation of the system implies the incentives within the system should be compatible with these structural components. If the incentives within the system are not compatible, then the incentives will have no effect on the system, or the system will not operate very smoothly, or the system must be changed to align with the incentives. For example, consider the case of creating a locally based food market. Farmers must have an incentive to participate in such a system, which would usually be the expectation of higher prices for their products. Consumers must also have an incentive to participate in the system, which may be the expectation of higher-quality products or a good feeling in terms of helping local farmers. In addition, the decision-making structure will often be designed or evolve to enhance the motivation structure and exploit the features of the information structure and vice versa. For example, in terms of a local farmers' market, farmers are more motivated to participate if they can set their own prices and consumers are more motivated to participate if they can negotiate on prices. Finally, the entire system will perform better the more transparent, easily accessed, and easily interpreted is the structure and data within the system. Establishing transparent guidelines and rules for qualifying as "local" food plus a transparent and reliable monitoring system assures consumers and producers that the market is what it claims to be: a local food market. Note that these three structural components interact and do not operate independently of each other. The more compatible these three components, the better the system will run. However, in a complex economic system consisting of many individuals or groups, many of the objectives within the system will be inconsistent and in conflict. As a result, there will be tradeoffs. Resolving conflict occurs one of two ways: domination or compromise. A system based on compromise is much more sustainable than a system based on domination. So in answering the six how, when, where, and whom questions, one must first understand the three core elements of an economic system.

Food systems can be quite complex, and further insights can be gained by appreciating that confirmation biases usually exist in evaluating a complex system. Different agents within the food or economic system will have different objectives that can lead to conflict, as is evident within the discussions of food systems (e.g., Freedhoff 2014; Stuckler and Nestle 2012; Yach 2014). At the heart of these debates is frequently some form of confirmation bias.

Recall from Chapter 9 that confirmation bias (effect) was defined as the tendency to search for, interpret, and use information to confirm a preconception and defend a choice. Two aspects of the food system exacerbate this cognitive bias. First, the inherent complexity of the food system and our individual limited cognitive power makes it impossible to understand all the components of the system in detail and therefore can lead to suspicion of the system or a fulfillment of the Roman proverb: "damnant quod non intelligent"—they condemn what they do not understand. Research suggests that learning about complex systems is difficult and that confirmation bias will be prevalent in a complex environment (Lehner at al. 2008; Sterman 1994). Second, the confirmation bias is also likely affected by intergroup bias. *Intergroup bias* is the systematic tendency to evaluate one's own membership group (the in-group) more favorably than a non-membership group (the out-group) (Hewstone, Rubin, and Willis 2002). Consequently, those in "nutrition groups" tend to view nutrition-based arguments and criticisms as more convincing than those in "industry groups," who view business arguments as more compelling.

What does all this imply? Humility is the first step to wisdom in understanding the food system and the different perspectives on that system. Reducing confirmation bias can be achieved by taking a more global view of the food system and in particular using several important principles from general systems theory (Bertalanffy 1979). The intuition of general systems theory is that analyzing system components in isolation will usually lead to faulty inferences and wrong conclusions. In systems theory, the whole is more than the sum of the parts. Here are five useful principles from systems theory to keep in mind when discussing food systems:

1. *Components of the system are interrelated.* Components generally do *not* operate independently (e.g., different food sectors).

2. *Systems are often dynamic.* The values of the variables within the system will change with time (e.g., quantities and prices).[3]

3. *There is usually feedback between system components.* Information is often transmitted in a bidirectional fashion between components within a system (e.g., consumers to food service providers to food processors to farmers and vice versa).

4. *The system will have some type of homeostasis.* Counteracting forces will tend to offset or at least attenuate the instability associated with a force considered in isolation (e.g., increasing prices help diminish demand for scarce products).

5. *Systems have an equifinality principle.* The outcome of a system can occur as the result of many influences and therefore in multiple ways (e.g., FAFH consumption may increase because of an increase in income or a decrease in time available for cooking at home).

The field of medicine provides a very good example where a system perspective is required for effective prevention and treatment, as the human body is clearly a complex system. For example, referred pain in the body occurs when pain in one location is due to a problem in another location. Classic examples of this are a heart attack manifesting as pain in the left arm or back pain due to problems with the pancreas. The physician who treats the location of the pain (the symptoms), not the sources of the pain (the cause), will be ineffective. The effective physician takes a systems perspective and can therefore identify the real source of the problem. In a similar fashion, to treat problems in the food system one must take a systems perspective to identify the real sources of the problem and how to address it within the mechanics of the system.

Think Break Questions

1. Given that the largest proportion of our food dollar does not go toward the food input, what are we actually buying when we purchase food (at home or away from home) within the U.S. food system?

2. What implication does your answer to Question 1 have for policies or interventions designed to change the food environment to support healthy eating?

3. Suppose you are working with a local extension agent to develop a local food market. Discuss why you may need to answer the six *what, how, how much, where, when,* and *for whom* questions before having an open meeting with farmers. Do you need to have answers to all of the questions or just some?

4. What confirmation bias might you suffer from in thinking about the food system as it relates to health?

---

[3] It should be quickly added that this does *not* mean the components or structure of the system change, only that the variables within the system are changing (e.g., think change in blood pressure in the human body system). Of course, one could change the system as well (e.g., add a pacemaker to the body), but that is now technically a different system.

5. How do the five principles from systems theory affect your view of the food environment?

Conclusions

This chapter gave an overview of the five major sectors in the U.S. food system and their contribution to the U.S. food dollar. The overview reveals that raw food products and ingredients constitute a minority of the value of inputs used in final consumer food products; the majority of the value is associated with marketing services. Deeper and broader insights come from recognizing that a food system is just a subsystem within an economic system, and all economic systems must answer six basic questions of production: *what, how, how much, where, when,* and *for whom* to produce. Each of these questions must be answered within each stage of the food system and within the motivation, decision-making, and information structure of the system. In evaluating these questions, the analyst who adheres to the six principles from systems theory is likely to provide more accurate and insightful suggestions for the functioning of the system than one who ignores these principles. So how are these questions answered in a production context? Let us cross the border and view the world from the producers' side.

Closing Conversation

JP: Wow. I didn't realize that the value of food had so little to do with food and was mostly marketing services. I also realize now that the food system is extremely complex and dynamic. How do food producers make decisions related to food production?

Margaret: Let's discuss that over dinner on Saturday. How about you bring the ingredients for a side dish and dessert and I'll make the main dish?

JP: Sounds good to me. But where are you getting your food from? And where would you recommend I buy my food? [wink wink]

12

Profit and Supply for Farms and Firms

Learning Objectives

What you will know by the end of this chapter:

- ¤ the importance of identifying the economic system setting;
- ¤ the definition of a firm and why firms exist;
- ¤ there is a lot of diversity across commodities and farm sizes in U.S. agriculture;
- ¤ the difference between economic profit and accounting profit;
- ¤ the tension and tradeoff between revenue and cost;
- ¤ the optimal location of output to maximize profit; and
- ¤ the difference between a firm's supply curve and its supply function.

Opening Conversation

JP [being greeted at the door by Margaret's dog, Honey]: Hi, Honey! How are you?

Margaret [answering JP]: Apparently our relationship has evolved to a new level. Hi, Honey! I'm fine.

JP: Ha! Well, there's often an element of truth in misstatements.

Margaret: Yes, there is. Did you also bring some honey for your dish?!

JP: Haha. I brought some fresh greens to make a salad and fruit for a dessert. I like to walk the talk, as you say, and eat healthfully. And speaking of these foods, how do farmers like those who grew these foods make production decisions?

Margaret: In short, they respond to market incentives. Let's start cooking and have a glass of wine and I can explain.

Setting the Stage for the Economics of Production

Chapter 11 gave an overview of economic systems that would apply to any economic system (e.g., capitalism, socialism, or communism). However, to identify the appropriate production objectives and incentives within a given system, the basic principles and boundaries of the economic system must first be understood.

While many may believe the United States is a capitalistic system, technically it is a mixed system. A *mixed economic system* allows for private economic freedom in the use of capital and the pursuit of profits, but only within the context of government regulations designed to promote some social aims. For example, food safety regulations are a government intervention designed to minimize health risks associated with foodborne illness. The standard approach to conducting an economic analysis, within a mixed system, is to start with a free market framework and then incorporate specific governmental policies or regulations as necessary to determine their effect. Indeed, we have already seen an example of this in Chapter 5, where we discussed the effects of a sugar-sweetened beverage tax. Even if not explicitly stated, the implicit assumption is that the consumers and producers in the market are obeying the laws and responding to the incentives that govern the particular market. Consequently, production will be driven mainly by a profit motive within the confines of the laws and incentives regulating the market.

Having identified the appropriate economic system context for U.S. food production, we must now be clear on the answer to two questions.

WHAT IS A FIRM?

A *firm* is an organization consisting of at least one person with the goal of producing a good to satisfy some objective. In economics the term *production* is the process of transforming resources and/or goods from one form, space, or time to another form, space, or time. This broad definition will cover obvious types of production, such as planting seeds to produce a crop, but will also include simple transportation, storage, repackaging, manufacturing, retailing, making a peanut butter sandwich at home, or doing a homework assignment. Furthermore, because labor is a resource, this definition includes not only goods (e.g., corn) but also services, such as nutrition education or medical services that are designed to produce something.

WHY DO FIRMS EXIST?

Some firms are small and some are large, but why do firms exist in the first place? In 1776, Adam Smith, the father of economics and author of *The Wealth of Nations* (Smith 1991), gave a classic example and answer. In Smith's day he noted a division of labor in a pin factory: one man draws out the wire, another straightens it, a third cuts it, a fourth points it, a fifth grinds it for receiving the head, another makes the head, another places the head on the pin, and so forth. Smith observed about 18 distinct operations involved in making a pin. He also observed that by such a division of labor, 10 low-skilled men could make about 48,000 pins per day, or

4,800 pins per man per day. How many pins could one man working alone make in a day? He would probably produce less than 100 and certainly nowhere near 4,800. By working together within a firm and by a division of labor (i.e., each doing a specialized tasks), the 10 men are able to make more pins than they could make separately working alone. What, then, determines the limit to this division of labor and the size of the firm? As Smith says (1991, Chapter 3. p. 15), "As it is the power of exchanging [consumers and producers engaging in transactions] so the extent of this division must always be limited by extent of that power, or, in other words, by the extent of the market. When the market is very small, no person can have any encouragement to dedicate himself entirely to one employment …"

What is the more general point of the pin (forgive the pun)? Firms exist because their organization is more efficient at producing some good than if the goods were produced without the organization, and their size is limited by their resources and the extent of the market for their goods. This is one reason why we have so many sectors involved in food production, because it is simply not very efficient and it is often infeasible for a single farm to grow food, process it, package it, transport it, and market it, as each one of these stages takes resources.

Against this backdrop, let's briefly look at some of the most important characteristics of farming in the United States before turning to the general economic principles of production.

Some Data on Farms

The United States has a total land area of about 2.3 billion acres. Farming acreage has remained constant at about 1 billion acres over the last century (Fig. 12.1). A century ago there were about 6.5 million farms in the United States and the

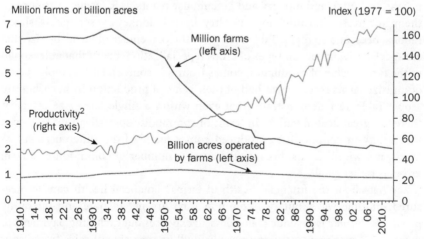

FIGURE 12.1 Farm Number, Acreage, and Productivity in United States, 1919-2013.

Source: Hoppe. Structure and Finances of US Farms: Family Farm Report. 2014. USDA.

U.S. population was about 100 million, so there were 15 people for every farm. However, today there are 150 people for every farm—a 10-fold increase—as the number of farms in the United States has drastically decreased over the last half-century.

While the acreage has remained relatively constant and the number of farms has decreased, farm output (productivity) has steadily increased. This amazing productivity increase has been due mainly to improvements in various technologies (e.g., seed varieties, breeding practices, tilling practices, pest and disease management). Few sectors in our economy have been as productive over a comparable period.

Given that a *farm* is any place where $1,000 or more of crops or livestock are sold, it should come as no surprise that farming in the United States is still mainly a family business. Farm size is classified by sales. *Small family farms* have sales of less than $350,000 in a year. *Midsize family farms* have sales between $350,000 and $999,999 in a year. *Large family farms* have sales greater than $1 million in a year. *Nonfamily farms* have no sales classification restriction. It is very tempting to conclude from these seemingly large numbers that farmers make a lot of money, but that is not true, as sales are not profit. You may sell your home for $150,000, but if you paid $200,000, you lost $50,000! We will look at the profitability of farming shortly. Table 12.1 gives the breakdown of the number of farms by size. Small farms make up about 90% of all farms, whereas large farms make up only about 2% of farms in the United States.

The diversity of commodities, which includes crops and livestock, produced in the United States is impressive. U.S. farmers grow wheat, oats, corn, soybeans, rice, grain sorghum, and other grains, such as rye, which are often called *cash grain crops*. *Other field crops* are crops such as cotton, peanuts, sugar beets, sugar cane, and tobacco.

High value crops refers to all the different fruits (e.g., strawberries, apples, blueberries), vegetables (e.g., carrots, potatoes, broccoli), tree nuts (e.g., pecans, walnuts), and nursery and greenhouse plants. U.S. farmers produce all the major livestock: cattle, hogs, poultry, horses, donkeys, bison, goats, sheep, rabbits, bees, and so forth. Table 12.1 gives the percentage of farms by size that are specializing in certain types of crops (specialization means that at least half of the farm's value of production comes from this source). For example, 54.5% of midsize farms receive over half of their value of production from cash grain crops. Table 12.1 demonstrates that even within a single farm size category, there is a great deal of variety in terms of commodity specialization. However, the variety in commodities produced comes mainly from differences across farms, not within farms, because the average number of commodities a farm grows is rather small.

What about the financial health of farms? Financial health can be measured multiple ways, but two common ways are net income and operating profit. *Net income* is revenue (sales) less all expenses but excluding payments to owners and management. *Farm revenues* will be the value of sales from crops and livestock plus government payments, and other farm-related income, like

TABLE 12.1

Number of Family Farms, Percentage Producing Selected Commodities, and Average Number of Commodities by Size, 2011[1]

	Small	Midsize	Large	Nonfamily	All
Number of Farms	1,949,261	123,009	42,398	58,175	2,172,843
Commodity Specialization[2]	Percentage				
Cash grain[3]	11.4	54.5	45.9	15.7	14.6
Other field crops[4]	23.6	7.7	10.3	27.3	22.6
High-value crops[5]	6.3	8.2	13.1	15.7	6.8
Beef	31.9	12.1	11.3	23.4	30.1
Hogs	0.6	2.8	4.6	1.4	0.8
Dairy	1.8	10.7	9.7	2.9	2.5
Poultry	2.5	2.2	2.8	1.1	2.4
Other livestock[6]	21.9	1.7	2.3	12.6	20.2
Average number of commodities	1.5	3.3	3.4	1.5	1.6

[1] Source: Hoppe. Structure and Finances of US Farms: Family Farm Report. 2014. USDA. Family farm size is classified based on gross cash farm income (GCFI). GCFI is the sum of the farm's crop and livestock sales, government payments, and other farm-related income. Small family farms have GCFI less than $350,000, midsize family farms have GCFI between $350,000 and $999,000, large family farms have GCFI over $1 million, and nonfamily farms have no criterion on GCFI. Data weighted and consolidated into small, midsize, and large by author.

[2] Commodity group accounts for at least half of farm's value of production.

[3] Includes wheat, corn, soybeans, grain sorghum, rice, and other general cash grains.

[4] Such as tobacco, peanuts, cotton, sugar beets, sugar cane, etc.

[5] Vegetables, fruits, tree nuts, nursery, greenhouse.

[6] Such as sheep, lambs, goats, horses, donkeys, rabbits, bees, bison, etc.

renting land to a neighboring farmer. *Farm expenses* are the cost of all inputs required to produce the crops and/or livestock. The main farm expenses are purchases of seed, livestock and poultry, feed, fertilizer, pesticides, fuel, electricity, machine hire (e.g., a tractor), repair services of equipment, marketing, storage, equipment, property taxes, hired labor (permanent), contract labor (temporary), and rent. *Operating profit* is net income less payments to operator labor and management. Operating profit is effectively the amount of money above what is required to pay all expenses, including the salary to the owner and management.

Figure 12.2 shows the percentage of farms in each size category that have a positive net farm income and a positive operating profit. Only 61% of small farms have a positive net income and only 30% have a positive operating profit. Coupling the data from Table 12.1 with that of Figure 12.2 indicates that most U.S. farms are not profitable (Hoppe 2014). These farms are able to stay in business by undervaluing their own labor in farming (i.e., they are effectively paying to farm) or by being subsidized by some form of off-farm income (e.g., an individual or spouse working in another job). What is clear from Figure 12.2 is that larger farms are more profitable than smaller farms, and this is mainly due to the lower cost of production per unit, something called *economies of size* in economics. The higher

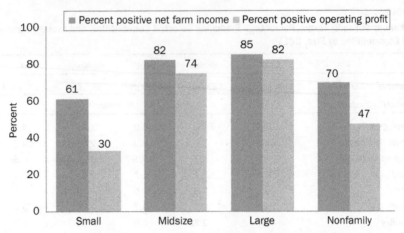

FIGURE 12.2 Percentage of Family Farms with Positive Net Farm Income and Positive Operating Profit by Family Farm Size, 2011.

Source: Hoppe. Structure and Finances of US Farms: Family Farm Report. 2014. USDA. Family farm size is classified based on gross cash farm income (GCFI). GCFI is the sum of the farm's crop and livestock sales, government payments, and other farm-related income. Small family farms have GCFI less than $350,000, midsize family farms have GCFI between $350,000 and $999,000, large family farms have GCFI over $1 million, and nonfamily farms have no criterion on GCFI. Net farm income is GCFI + net inventory change + home consumption + imputed value of farm dwelling – cash expenses – noncash benefits for paid labor – depreciation. Operating profit is net farm income + interest paid – charge for operator and unpaid labor – charge for management. Data weighted and consolidated into small, midsize, and large by authors.

profitability is generally not because they receive more for each unit sold. Let's now turn to the general economics of production and profitability.

Paul's Potato Production and Profit

Though there is great variety in the number of commodities produced and the size of farm operations, the underlying production economic principles are the same regardless of enterprise. Consequently, the rest of the chapter focuses on these principles. Much like the consumer case, production decisions are multidimensional (e.g., multiple inputs are used to produce an output). To solidify the foundations, we start with a simple case where one input (labor) is being used to harvest a crop.

Paul is a potato farmer and ready to harvest his crop. Where he lives, potatoes are harvested by hand. Paul wants to know how many men he should hire to harvest potatoes to maximize his profit. Where he lives, Paul knows the current wage rate per hour for harvesting potatoes is $8 and a bushel of potatoes sells for $3. Table 12.2 gives the data associated with the number of workers (input), bushels harvested, costs, revenues, and profits on a per-hour basis.

Notice what happens in the second column to the number of bushels harvested per hour as the number of workers hired increases. The first worker

TABLE 12.2
Paul's Potato Production, Cost, Revenue and Profit Per Hour Example

Workers (number)	Potatoes (bushels)	Total Cost (TC)	Total Revenue (TR)	Profit (TR – TC)
0	0	0	0	0
1	2	8	6	–2
2	8	16	24	8
3	18	24	54	30
4	24	32	72	40
5	25	40	75	35
6	18	48	54	6

harvests 2 bushels per hour. Adding a second worker increases the harvest to 8 bushels an hour. Adding a third worker increases the harvest to 18 bushels an hour, the fourth to 24 bushels an hour, and the fifth to 25 bushels an hour. But adding the sixth worker decreases the harvest back to 18 bushels an hour. What is going on?

This type of production pattern is common where there are at first *increasing returns to scale* (i.e., output increases faster than inputs) and then *decreasing returns to scale* (i.e., output increases at a slower rate than inputs). We discussed this type of pattern in the consumer case of health production. There are many possible reasons why this type of pattern may occur. Some of the increase in productivity may have been in organizational efficiency coming from a division of labor as in the pin factory, such as designating some of the workers just to unload and retrieve empty baskets. The key is that at some point these efficiency gains per worker begin to decrease after a certain number of workers (e.g., four workers). This could be due to the "too many cooks in the kitchen" phenomenon, where there is simply not much for the fifth worker to do or he is actually interfering with work.

Columns 3, 4, and 5 give the total cost, the total revenue from selling what was harvested, and then the total profit per hour, respectively. With labor as the only input, total cost is the price per unit of labor per hour ($8) times the number of workers hired. Total revenue is the price that Paul can sell a bushel of potatoes for ($3) times the number of bushels harvested. *Profit* is the difference between total revenue and total cost. Paul is looking for the point where the difference in total revenue and total cost is the greatest or profit is maximized. Note this occurs where output is 24 bushels per hour or four workers are hired (the shaded row). Profit is *not* maximized where output is greatest or revenue is greatest (i.e., five workers, 25 bushels per hour, $75 in revenue) because those numbers in isolation ignore cost and cost is also higher at five workers (i.e., $40). Furthermore, profit is *not* maximized where cost would be the least, which would be at zero workers and bushels. This is a key take-home message, which we will repeat again and again: One must look at revenues and cost when discussing profit. *Profit is maximized where the difference between total revenue and total cost is greatest.*

The Economics of Profit: Total Revenue Minus Total Cost

We can gain greater insights by expressing the definition of profit succinctly in a math paragraph:

$$Profit = TR(y, p) - TC(y, r_1, r_2, ..., r_n): \ Profit \qquad (12.1)$$

where TR denotes total revenue, y is output, p is the price per unit p, and TC denotes total cost, which depends on the output y and the prices of the different inputs r_1, r_2...,r_n. We are now including the prices of many (all) inputs and the profit equation is not limited to just two inputs.

Let's first think about these components separately and start with total cost. $TC(y, r_1, r_2, ..., r_n)$ is the *total cost function* and represents the *minimum* cost required to produce the quantity of the output y. Minimizing the cost of producing a given output y will imply that the firm is looking for the optimal combination of inputs to reach a given output level at minimum cost. Maximizing profit by definition then implies cost minimization. Why? Consider Paul's potato farm again. To produce 24 bushels of potatoes requires four workers and costs $32. Paul can sell 24 bushels for $3 per bushel, or $72 in total revenue. His profit is $40. Now suppose Paul figures out a way to produce those 24 bushels with only three workers. In this case, his revenue has not changed and is still $72, but his total cost is now $24 (three workers), so now his profit is $48, which is $8 more than he was making. So, by definition, he was not maximizing profit before. Consequently, maximizing profit can be thought of as occurring in two stages. In the first stage, the firm is simply trying to figure out how to produce a given level of output as efficiently as possible.[1]

There are two types of costs, which are associated with two types of inputs: fixed and variable. *Total fixed cost* (*TFC*) refers to the sum of all costs that *do not* vary with output, such as the number of tractors or acres a farmer has on his farm. *Total variable cost* (*TVC*) refers to the sum of all costs that *do vary* with output, such as the tractor fuel or labor hours required for planting and harvesting. Thus the total cost component of Equation 12.1 can be written as

$$TC = TFC + TVC(y, r_1, r_2, ..., r_n): \ Total \ cost \ decomposition \qquad (12.2)$$

Let's now consider the revenue part of the profit equation. If the firm faces a fixed price for its output, it is considered a *price taker*. A firm can be a price taker for many reasons. It may simply have no power to demand a higher price in the market. For example, if the potato processing plant that buys Paul's potatoes can buy potatoes from other farmers, then if Paul tries to charge a higher price for his

---

[1] Most economics books for majors will have one or two chapters on production and cost minimization, which is the first stage of profit maximization (e.g., Varian 2006). We do not include the details of this first stage so that we can focus more on the ultimate economic issue of the tradeoff between revenues and costs.

potatoes, the processing plant can say, "Sorry, I don't have to pay that price because your sister Mary down the road will sell them to me for a cheaper price." There is a sufficient supply in the market, so the processing plant can buy enough from another source.[2] Alternatively, Paul may have negotiated a contractual price with the processing plant prior to harvesting his crop. The main point is the price is the same for all units sold. In this context, the total revenue component of Equation 12.1 can be written as

$$TR(y,p) = p \times y : \text{ Total revenue for price taker} \qquad (12.3)$$

Let's now put all this back together by substituting Equations 12.3 and 12.2 into Equation 12.1 to get

$$Profit = p \times y - TFC - TVC(y, r_1, r_2, ..., r_n) : \text{ Profit decomposition} \qquad (12.4)$$

So from Equation 12.4, profit can vary depending on the price of the output (p), the amount sold (y), the total fixed cost (TFC), and the total variable cost (TVC), which depends on how much is produced and how much is paid for the inputs (i.e., the variable input prices).

Before proceeding, we need to be clear on an important point: *economic profit is not the same as accounting profit. Accounting profit* refers to the amount of revenue in excess of the *market costs* associated with *all* factors of production. *Economic profit* refers to the amount of revenue in excess of the *opportunity costs* of *all* factors of production. What is the difference? As we have already discussed earlier in the book, opportunity cost refers to the cost of forgoing the next best alternative. In the production context it would refer to the next best alternative use of inputs used in production. For example, Paul's potato farm makes an accounting profit of $40 per hour when he employs four workers. However, this is not his economic profit. Paul's economic profit is something less than $40 because Paul has an opportunity cost for running his farm. Suppose Paul could work for his sister Mary managing her potato farm for $30 an hour. Taking into account Paul's opportunity cost, his economic profit from running his own farm is then $40 – $30 = $10 per hour. So after paying himself his opportunity cost (i.e., his market wage rate), he still has $10 extra to do with what he wants, so he is better off running his own potato farm than working for his sister Mary. Accounting profit is the profit shown on the books, whereas economic profit will be accounting profit less the opportunity cost of inputs, so accounting profit will be greater than economic profit. This explains why the percentage of farms with positive net farm income (an accounting concept) was higher than the percentage of farms with positive operating profit (an economic concept) in Figure 12.2. The main input whose opportunity cost is not captured by the market price of the input is usually the

---

[2] We will discuss in more detail market structures in Chapter 14.

owner's labor time.[3] The total cost in Equation 12.2 and 12.4 are considered inclusive of opportunity cost.

So how do we determine the optimal output that maximizes profit? There are two approaches, the total approach and the per unit approach, each leading to the same answer. Both of these approaches are useful for different reasons, so let's consider each.

THE TOTAL APPROACH TO DETERMINING OPTIMAL OUTPUT

The optimal output level will occur where the difference in total revenue and total cost is greatest. What does this look like graphically? Figure 12.3 shows the total revenue and total cost curves in general for a price-taking firm.

The vertical axis intercept for the total cost curve is the total fixed cost (*TFC*), as this is the cost that is incurred even with no production. Increasing output requires purchasing more inputs, so total cost (*TC*) will increase as output increases. The *TC* does not usually increase in a constant (linear) fashion because at first the firm is trying to figure out the most efficient production methods, so cost may increase rather rapidly. However, once the firm has a system and a set of fixed resources in place, the owners are likely able to increase output over a range without a great increase in total cost as they exploit efficiencies with their firm. However, at some point they start to run up against limits of efficiency exploitation, due perhaps to technological constraints or labor skill constraints or other input constraints (e.g., the fertility of the soil), and the cost of additional output increases greatly. All these stages were seen in Paul's potato farm. This is the most general shape of the total cost curve and it represents all the relevant possibilities for the shape of the total cost curve. Different firms will have different total cost curves. For some firms some segments will cover a wider range of output and some segments will cover a shorter range of output.

So what is happening to profit in Figure 12.3? When output is between zero and point *B*, profit is actually negative because total revenue is *less than* total cost (*TR* < *TC*). Point *B* corresponds to the "break-even" output level because total revenue is exactly covering total cost (*TR* = *TC*). After point *B*, profit becomes positive and increases as total revenue is increasing faster than total cost, until y^* is reached. Profit is maximized at the optimal output level y^* and the profit level is Profit* = TR* − TC*. In the case of Paul's potato farm, the optimal output occurred at 24 bushels per hour for a profit of $40 per hour.

Importantly, note that if the total fixed cost (*TFC*) were higher, the total cost curve would have a higher intercept, so the total cost curve would shift up.

---

[3] Economic profit does not include the psychic benefits (or costs) associated with running a business. If there is psychic income (utility), then it is completely possible for a firm to show a negative accounting and economic profit and yet still be in operation, at least in the short run or if subsidized by some other activity. For example, it is not uncommon to see farmers with negative farm accounting profits who subsidize their farming operations with off-farm income because they just enjoy farming. Succinctly stated, they are willing to pay to farm, as was discussed regarding the numbers in Figure 12.2

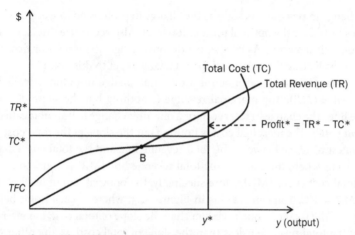

FIGURE 12.3 Optimal Output for Greatest Total Profit.
[IAPS] Total profit is greatest when the difference between total revenue and total cost is greatest, which occurs at y*.

Alternatively, if the price of some variable input increases, each unit of output would cost more to produce and the total cost curve would rotate counterclockwise. Also, if the price of the output increased, then the total revenue line would rotate counterclockwise as well.

THE PER UNIT APPROACH TO DETERMINING OPTIMAL OUTPUT

Our ultimate interest is to determine how output will change as the price of the output in the market changes or the cost of production changes. This is more easily achieved by thinking in terms of profit per unit of output and the *change in profit* as output changes.

The intuition behind the change in profit focus is more easily seen with the math sentence

$$\Delta Profit = \Delta Total\,Revenue - \Delta Total\,Cost > 0:$$
$$\textit{Produce / sell more condition} \tag{12.5}$$

where Δ is shorthand notation for change. Note that Equation 12.5 implies $\Delta Total\,Revenue > \Delta Total\,Cost$: the change in total revenue is greater than the change in cost. More money is being made than is being spent, so the profit-maximizing producer should keep increasing production until

$$\Delta Profit = \Delta Total\,Revenue - \Delta Total\,Cost = 0:$$
$$\textit{Optimal production condition} \tag{12.6}$$

Don't let this simple math throw you. In practice a farmer would simply start changing his production level and note the change in costs and then compare this to the change in revenue. As soon as the change in profit is no longer positive, this indicates he is near the optimal production level. Also recognize this is *not* a static condition; it is dynamic. As market conditions change, the farmer or firm is continuously evaluating this relationship and trying to get to this point.

The change in total revenue for a one-unit change in output is called *marginal revenue (MR)*. The marginal revenue is nothing but the slope of the total revenue line. The change in total cost for a one-unit change in output is called *marginal cost (MC)*. The marginal cost is nothing but the slope of the total cost curve. The greatest distance between the total revenue line and the total cost curve will always occur where the slope of the total revenue line (MR) is equal to the slope of the total cost curve (MC). More succinctly, the optimal output level y^* occurs where $MR = MC$. You can see this in Figure 12.3, where at each point before y^* the slope of the total revenue is greater than the slope of total cost, but after y^* the slope of the total revenue is less than the slope of total cost. At any other output level, the distance between total revenue and total cost will not be as great. Note that because the firm is a price taker and the total revenue line has a constant slope equal to the price of the output, then we further have the condition $MR = p$. So the optimal output level y^* for a price-taking firm occurs where

$$p = MC : Profit\ maximization\ condition\ for\ a\ price\text{-}taking\ firm \qquad (12.7)$$

The graph of the profit-optimizing condition $p = MC$ turns out to be a critical element in showing how the firm's output will change as the price in the market changes. However, to complete the per unit analysis we also need to know something about average total cost. By incorporating average total cost, we will be able to show the breakeven point analogous to point B in Figure 12.3, and we will also be able to show the profit level, similar to Figure 12.3.

The *average total cost (ATC)* of production is just the total cost divided by total output, so it is just the average cost per unit produced. Consequently, simply divide both sides of Equation 12.2 by y or

$$ATC = \frac{TC}{y} = \frac{TFC}{y} + \frac{TVC}{y} = AFC + AVC \qquad (12.8)$$

So average total cost per unit produced (ATC) has an average fixed cost (AFC) component and an average variable cost (AVC) component.

The entire per unit analysis can now be captured graphically (Fig. 12.4). All of the cost curves are decreasing over some range before they start to increase. As in the total cost case, these shapes are associated with the different returns to scale. To simplify the graph, we have not shown the average fixed cost (AFC), but recognize that because $ATC = AFC + AVC$, the *area* between the ATC curve and the AVC curve is equal to AFC. It is a technical fact to just remember that the marginal cost (MC) curve will always intersect the ATC curve and the AVC curve at their lowest points. As explained, the profit maximization output y^* will occur where $p = MC$. Take note that because $ATC = TC/y$, then $TC = ATC \times y$. Furthermore, we know

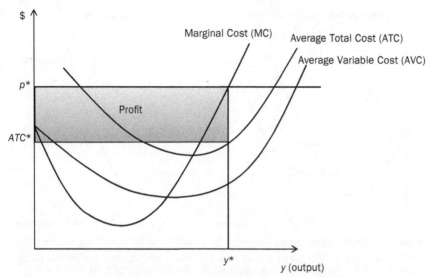

FIGURE 12.4 Optimal Output for Greatest Total Profit from Marginal Analysis.
[IAPS] Total profit is greatest at the output level $y*$ where the marginal cost is equal to the price of the output.

$TR = p \times y$, so we have the very useful relationship $Profit = TR - TC = (p - ATC) \times y$. The amount of profit is therefore shown by the shaded rectangle labeled "profit" and is equal to $(p - ATC*) \times y*$. The term $(p - ATC)$ can be thought of as profit margin per unit sold.

The Firm's Supply

One of the main reasons for understanding the economics of profit maximization is to determine how the quantity supplied of a good will change as market conditions change, such as the cost of inputs or the price of the output. Similar to the consumer demand curves and functions in Chapter 5, we now want to derive the individual firm's supply curve and relate it to the firm's supply function.

THE FIRM'S SUPPLY CURVE

The *firm's supply curve* shows the relationship between the firm's optimal output level and the price received for the output. There is a close relationship between the firm's supply curve and its marginal cost curve, as shown in Figure 12.5. Consider the left panel. When the price is anything less than p_0, the optimal quantity supplied by the firm is zero. Why? Because at any price less than p_0, the average variable cost (AVC) will be greater than the price, which simply means the firm cannot even pay for all its variable inputs required to grow and harvest the crop (e.g., labor, fuel, fertilizer). At the price p_0 and output y_0, the firm is making exactly enough money to pay for the variable inputs, so y_0 is known as the *shutdown point*.

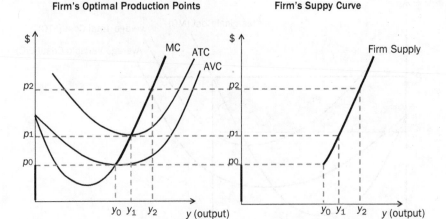

FIGURE 12.5 Firm's Optimal Output Production and Supply Curve for an Increase in Output Price. [IAPS] The firm's supply curve shows how the firm's output changes as the price of the output changes and is the same as the firm's marginal cost above the average variable cost curve.

As the price increases above p_0, then production increases according to the marginal cost curve because of the optimization condition $p = MC$.

Importantly, between p_0 and p_1, the firm's owners are *not* making a positive profit, but they are making more than the cost of their variable inputs, so they are in the market. They can pay some money toward their fixed cost but they cannot cover all of their fixed cost. For example, suppose Paul bought four used hoes off eBay for harvesting potatoes for $20. When Paul hired two workers he had to pay them $16, but he made $24, so he was making $8 over his variable labor cost. This extra $8 could be put toward the $20 he paid for the hoes, but he still owes $12 on the hoes. So more generally, any price between p_0 and p_1 is sufficient to cover the variable input cost, but not also all of the fixed input cost.

The price p_1 and quantity y_1 is known as the *breakeven point* because at this point total revenue (*TR*) exactly equals total cost (*TC*), so the economic profit is zero, which is easily seen by writing profit in its alternative form $(p - ATC) \times y$. This point corresponds to point *B* in Figure 12.3. Any price above p_1 implies a positive profit and the firm's supply curve is its marginal cost curve.

Putting all this logic together, the right-hand panel shows the firm's supply curve, which is just the collection of all optimal price/quantity combinations that maximize profit, *ceteris paribus*. Each quantity point on the supply curve represents a specific *quantity supplied* (e.g., 24 bushels of potatoes). Furthermore, each price point on the supply curve represents the minimum amount the firm is willing and able to accept for that quantity supplied. A *movement along the supply curve is a change in quantity supplied.*

As different firms will have different cost curves, they will also have different supply curves. Some firms are able to respond to a change in output price at a greater rate than some other firms. In this case the slopes of their supply curves will be different, as shown in Figure 12.6. Suppose both firms are receiving the

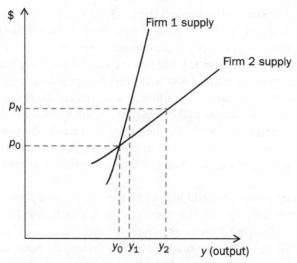

FIGURE 12.6 Different Firms with Different Supply Curves.
[IAPS] Firm 1 has a more elastic (responsive) supply curve than Firm 1.

price p_0 and therefore both have the optimal output y_0. Suppose now the price increases to a new price, p_N. Firm 1 is able to increase output only to y_1, whereas Firm 2 is able to increase output to y_2. This difference could be for many possible reasons, such as Firm 2 simply has more productive land, or more productive workers, or a better management system. Similar to the consumer case, we use the term *supply elasticity* to refer to the percentage change in output for a percentage change in the price of the output. If the supply elasticity is less than 1, then supply is said to be *inelastic*. If the supply elasticity is greater than 1, then supply is said to be *elastic*.

The steeper the supply curve, then the less elastic it will be, so in Figure 12.6, Firm 1 has a more inelastic supply curve than Firm 2. If the supply curve is a vertical line, then it is said to be *perfectly inelastic*, and if the supply curve is a horizontal line, it is said to be *perfectly elastic*.

THE FIRM'S SUPPLY CURVE VERSUS THE SUPPLY FUNCTION

Similar to the demand curve discussion in Chapter 5, the term *supply curve* here is reserved for showing a two-dimensional relationship between the quantity supplied by the firm and the price received for its output on the market, *ceteris paribus*. As in the consumer case, economics recognizes that other factors may affect the quantity supplied by the firm, and the main other factors are input prices. The firm's *supply function* is the general multidimensional representation of the firm's quantity supply response to changes in important factors and is written as

$$y = y(P, r_1, r_2, v): \textit{Firm's supply function} \qquad (12.9)$$
$${\scriptstyle (+)\ (-)\ (-)\ (?)}$$

As in Chapter 5, this math paragraph succinctly tells us (a) what variables affect quantity supplied and (b) the direction of their effect. As before, the paragraph is read as the quantity supplied of y depends positively on its own price p, negatively on the price of inputs r_1 and r_2 (only two are shown, but there may be more), and an unknown or unspecified way with other factors v. So the supply curve in Figure 12.6 captures the first relationship by a movement along the curve, given that price is on the vertical axis. The change in any other variable (i.e., r_1, r_2, or v) will be represented by a shift in the supply curve (i.e., for the same price, less or more would be produced). A shift in the supply curve is sometimes simply called a change in supply, which should be distinguished from a change in quantity supplied.

Figure 12.7 shows what will happen to the supply curve if the price of, say, Input 1 (r_1) increases. As the price of an input increases, this will cause the marginal cost of production for each unit to increase, which in turn will cause the supply curve to shift up (or for the same price shift to the left), as shown in Figure 12.7. How far the supply curve shifts is determined by how much the price increased and the degree of substitution between the inputs. A larger price increase or fewer substitutes will lead to a greater shift.

Master Manipulator

1. Using Figure 12.4, show what happens to the graph if the price of the output decreased. What would happen to the optimal level of output in this case?
2. Using Figure 12.4 as your guide, show what will happen to the marginal, average total, and average variable cost of production of potatoes if the

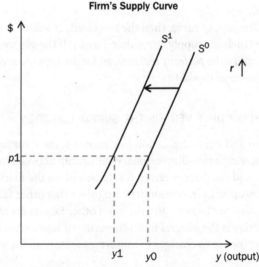

Firm's Supply Curve

FIGURE 12.7 Decrease in a Firm's Supply if the Price of an Input Increases.
[IAPS] The firm's supply curve shifts if an input price changes.

price of tractor fuel increases. What will happen to the optimal output level and the level of profit?

3. What would happen to the supply curve in Figure 12.7 if immigration laws were relaxed such that the price of farm labor decreased? Relating this back to Figure 12.4, what do you think will happen to profit in this case?

Conclusions

We have covered a lot of material here rather concisely. In Chapter 11, we indicated there were six questions that all economies must answer in terms of production: what, how, how much, where, when, and for whom to produce. The profit objective covered in this chapter provides a framework for answering all of these questions within a mixed economic system. The reader should start to appreciate the importance of the tradeoffs a firm will face when selling a good, and often that tradeoff is between revenues and costs. Any recommendations about what farms should produce (e.g., organic foods) need to address *both* sides of the profit calculation to be realistic and feasible.

If a certain type of food, such as "certified organic" apples, costs more to produce, perhaps due to more susceptibility to disease or pests, then to ensure a positive profit, the revenue from the product must be higher. This means the selling price must be higher before the producer would even consider growing an organic product. When considering the production of alternative commodities, great insights will usually come from first just comparing the differences in revenues *and* costs between the alternatives. Two crops may have similar prices, but if the second has a lower cost of production, then there is an incentive to produce and sell that crop. Alternatively, if one crop costs more to produce, then this is a disincentive for producing this crop—unless consumers are willing to pay a higher price for that product.

All of the concepts presented in this chapter apply for all types of firms, from farmers to multinational companies. Consequently, with this background we can quickly expand on these concepts in the next chapter by looking at profit maximization in a more general setting that may apply beyond the farm gate.

Closing Conversation

JP: Geez. That is almost as intricate as the consumer side. However, it is rather intuitive. I always realized that if a farmer had a choice between growing an organic peach versus a non-organic peach, he would have to look not only at the revenue but also the cost. However, what this helped me realize was that it's not enough that the price of organic peaches be higher, it must be high enough to completely offset the higher cost.

Margaret: Exactly! [Looking at her dog Honey] Would you like a glass of wine, Honey?

JP: I don't mind if I do.

Margaret [Laughing]: You started it.

13

Production and Profit Beyond the Farm Gate

Learning Objectives

What you will know by the end of this chapter:

¤ the connection between downstream and upstream firms;
¤ the implications of profit maximization for price-taking and price-making firms;
¤ how market segmentation affects the distribution of healthy and unhealthy foods;
¤ the definition of corporate social responsibility;
¤ the implications of corporate social responsibility for profit maximization; and
¤ why strategic corporate responsibility may be difficult.

Opening Conversation

JP [on phone to Margaret]: Margaret! Hey, I have two tickets to a concert for Honey and the Bees next Saturday. Would you like to go?

Margaret: Yeah.

JP: Great. I'll pick you up at 7:30. I hope you don't mind if I ask you some more questions about the production side of the food market anyway.

JP [on the way to the concert]: OK, here are the questions. Last time you talked about maximizing profit but assumed the firms could not set their own prices. That seems like a strong assumption. Plus, I'm curious about the economics, or tradeoffs, a food processing firm like Kraft faces between making profits and facing negative publicity by consumer advocacy groups who say they are contributing to obesity, for example. It would seem that bad publicity could affect their profits.

Margaret: Wow, that's a lot. This could be a late night!

Introduction

This chapter focuses on the economics of production for any firms in the supply chain that are beyond the farm gate: the food marketing sector. This *food marketing sector* consists of all farm raw product wholesalers, food and beverage manufacturers, food wholesalers, and food retailers. As shown in Chapter 11, these firms account for the largest percentage of the food dollar, but profitability varies quite significantly within this sector. For example, in 2012 farm product raw product wholesalers averaged revenues about 10% above expenses, whereas food and beverage stores had revenues about 28% above expenses (U.S. Census Bureau, Business and Industry 2015). However, the fundamental profitability concepts are the same regardless of whether a firm sells organic apples at a farmers' market or roasted chickens in a grocery store. This chapter extends the analysis of Chapter 12 in three directions.

First, to understand the economics of the food system, the sectors in the food system must be connected via input and output prices through the profit analysis. Second, as one approaches the retail end of the supply chain, some firms are able to charge different prices at different levels of output. In this case, the profit analysis must be extended to the price maker case. Finally, there is a lot of debate about the contribution of the food industry to the nutritional quality of our food supply, so we want to provide a framework for analyzing the important issue of corporate social responsibility (CSR) in the food industry.

The Downstream Price-Taking Firm

In economic terminology, the five food sectors in the marketing channel are vertically linked. Raw farm and fishing products are sold to farm raw product wholesalers, which sell to food and beverage manufacturers, which sell to food wholesalers, which sell to food retailers. The terms "downstream firm" and "upstream firm" are often used to understand the links. A firm is *downstream* in the marketing channel if it uses inputs from another (*upstream*) firm in the marketing channel. If Firm 1 sells its products to Firm 2, then Firm 1 is the upstream firm and Firm 2 is the downstream firm.

The price-taking downstream firm faces the same type of economic problem the farm-level firm faced in Chapter 12, so we can write profit as

$$\text{Profit} = p \times y - TC(y, r_1, r_2, ..., r_n): \text{ Profit decomposition} \qquad (13.1)$$

The variables p, y, and r_1, r_2,...,r_n refer to the price, output, and input prices *for the firm or food sector being discussed.* For a wholesaler shipping strawberries, y and p may refer to the quantity and price per pallet of strawberries and the relevant input prices r may be the fuel costs and labor costs associated with transporting the strawberries 300 miles. Alternatively, for a food processor selling ice cream, y and p may refer to the quantity and price per gallon of ice cream and the relevant input prices r may be labor costs or ingredient costs, such as strawberries.

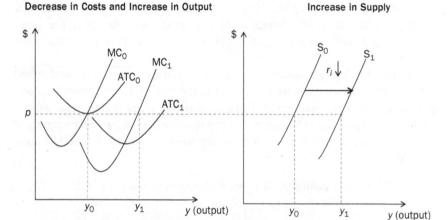

FIGURE 13.1 Marketing Sector Firm's Change in Costs and Supply as an Input Price Decreases. [IAPS] As the price of an input to the marketing service firm decreases, the firm's cost curves shift down as cost decreases, the output level increases, and consequently the supply curve shifts to the right.

Figure 13.1 shows what will happen if the price of an input in the food marketing sector decreases. This should look familiar. All of the logic from Figure 12.8 applies here too, so we can be brief.

As the price of some input r_i decreases, the original average and marginal cost curves (ATC_0, MC_0) shift down (or to the right) because the cost per unit has decreased to, say, ATC_1 and MC_1. The output price p has not decreased for the firm because it is a price taker, so the profit-maximizing output, where $p = MC$, increases from y_0 to y_1 and correspondingly the supply curve shifts out from S_0 to S_1. The general concepts captured by Figure 13.1 apply to any type of firm in the food marketing channel. The key difference from Chapter 12 is that the input price that has changed for the downstream firm is the output price for an upstream firm. For example, the price received by strawberry farmers (the upstream firm) is the price paid for strawberries by the raw farm product wholesaler (the downstream firm).

The Downstream Price-Making Firm

In many cases, the firm may be able to adjust the price of its product within a certain feasible range determined by competition within the market.[1] This is especially true the closer one gets to the final consumer for many food items because as one moves away from the farm toward the consumer, the products become more differentiated and thus there is less competition. Major quick-service national chain restaurants like Panera or Wendy's certainly choose the selling prices for their sandwiches (e.g., $6), but competition with other restaurants prevents them

---

[1] Different types of competition will be discussed in Chapter 14.

from setting *any* price they want (e.g., $12). They are price makers, but they are constrained by the law of demand: as the price of the good increases, the quantity demanded decreases, *ceteris paribus*, because there are other competing goods available.

To handle the price making case, all we have to do is substitute the demand function in for every place we had output in the profit formula above. Let's add one more realistic component. A firm may also alter other attributes (*a*) associated with the food in an attempt to increase revenue (e.g., sugar, fat, background music, or even advertising). Let's therefore write the demand function quite generally as

$$y = y(\underset{-\ +}{p,a}): \text{Demand for the good with certain attributes} \tag{13.2}$$

Recall that the little negative sign under the price indicates that as the price increases, *less* is sold (law of demand), *ceteris paribus*. Similarly, the little positive sign under *a* indicates that as the attribute *a* is increased, the demand for the good increases, *ceteris paribus*.[2] Of course, we could have a case where increasing an attribute decreased the demand, but the impact will simply be the opposite of that discussed here.

Substituting Equation 13.2 into 13.1 gives the more general profit relationship

$$Profit = p \times y(\underset{-\ +}{p,a}) - TC\left[\underset{-\ +\ +\ +\ +}{y(p,a),a,r_1,r_2}\right]: \tag{13.3}$$

Price making profit w / other attributes

There are three separate price effects on profit now. Let's read this paragraph from left to right with respect to price. The first effect of increasing the price would make each unit sold (*y*) more valuable. The second effect of increasing the price, however, decreases the amount sold, via the law of demand. The third effect of increasing the price actually decreases the cost because as the amount sold decreases due to the law of demand, less is produced, so total cost would decrease as well. So increasing the price has positive and negative impacts on profit. The ultimate question is: Where should the price be set to maximize profit?

Figure 13.2 is a generalized version of Figure 12.4 from Chapter 12. Consider the total revenue (*TR*) curve. As the price of the good is increased, total revenue at first will be increasing as the increase in price is greater than the decrease in the quantity demanded. But at some point the decrease in the quantity demanded will be greater than the price increase, so total revenue will begin to decrease. As the quantity produced (sold) increases, the total cost (*TC*) is increasing as well. Profit will be maximized again where the distance between total revenue and total cost

---

[2] For simplicity, we are ignoring other factors, such as income or substitute prices, that are not controlled by the firm, but they certainly affect demand as well.

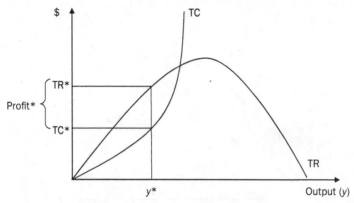

FIGURE 13.2 Profit Maximization Output with Price-Making Firm.

is the greatest, at y_*.[3] Except where the total cost of production is zero, profit is *not* maximized where total revenue is maximized.

Let's now explore a case where a firm is considering adjusting one of the attributes of a food. For example, recently Chipotle, the Mexican-food chain, decided to switch to tortillas made from organic, unbleached, and unenriched flour. As Chipotle indicates, this is expected to increase its cost (Newsday 2015).

Figure 13.3 and Equation 13.3 help us understand the tradeoff the chain may face.

The initial total revenue and total cost associated with the original tortillas are represented by TR_0 and TC_0 respectively, along with the optimal output of y_0 and the profit denoted by the gray area. Because the new tortillas are more expensive, the cost per unit of output will increase and the cost curve would rotate counterclockwise to TC_1. If nothing else changed (the total revenue curve did not change), the price of the product would be increased to offset the cost increase, and by the law of demand this would decrease the quantity demanded. The profit-maximizing quantity would decrease and profits would decrease. However, the only real reason a firm would consider using a more expensive input is if it felt demand would increase (shift out) because of the new healthier ingredients. So on the revenue side, we will assume that switching to the organic tortilla may also increase the demand for the food item even at the higher price, so the total revenue curve would rotate counterclockwise as well to TR_1. Profit is still maximized where the distance between total revenue and total cost is the greatest, now at y_1. As we have drawn this example, the new profit (dark-shaded area) with the organic tortillas is smaller than the profit with the original tortillas, so the original tortillas are more profitable.

Note from Figure 13.3 that to increase profit, it is not enough that the total revenue curve shifts up. The increase in revenue must be greater than the increase in cost.

---

[3] As in Chapter 12, one could express the profit-maximization condition in terms of the marginal conditions. However, the main intuition we want to obtain is available from the total graph presented here.

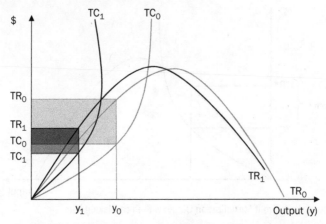

FIGURE 13.3 Change in Profit-Maximizing Output with a Greater Increase in Cost than Revenue due to an Attribute Change.
[IAPS] Profit and output may decrease even though demand for the product increased if the increase in cost is greater than the increase in revenue.

Many other possibilities could be drawn. By deciding to switch to organic tortillas, Chipotle believes that revenue will increase (shift up) enough to offset the cost increase, so profits would increase, which certainly may happen. The main point to remember is that profit can change because (1) only revenue changed, (2) only cost changed, or (3) some combination. A complete analysis requires discussing the change in revenue *and* cost.

Some Profitable Exercises

1. As indicated, Chipotle certainly believes going to organic tortillas will increase revenues more than cost, so that profits will increase. Draw a figure similar to Figure 13.3 but where profit increased instead of decreased. Does the optimal output have to increase in this case?
2. List some reasons why you think the total revenue would be *greater* or the total cost would be *less* for healthy foods. Explain your economic reasoning. Do you have any evidence for or against this position?

The Distribution of Unhealthy and Healthy Foods from a Production Perspective

The distribution of foods in the United States is skewed toward "unhealthy" foods—foods high in sugar, sodium, fat, and calories, especially for food away from home (e.g., Hearst et al. 2013; Lin and Guthrie 2012; Poti et al. 2015; Wu 2015; Wu and Sturm 2013). Does this evidence imply that unhealthy foods are more profitable than healthy foods? Not categorically; one can selectively find support on both sides of the argument.

In stark contrast to consumer research, very little research exists asking producers why they offer certain foods. In the dearth of published research, interviewed executives cite higher cost and a lack of an increase in demand as the main reasons healthier options are not offered, implying they are less profitable (e.g., Glanz et al. 2007; Obbagy et al. 2011). Jonathan Marek, senior vice president of Applied Predictive Technologies, a company that helps companies predict expenses and profitability initiatives, states it this way: "[As restaurants shift toward healthier menus, operators will] need to see a lift in sales in order to pay out the additional costs on the sourcing of better products . . . Everything has cost implications, but it is primarily about the demand [revenue] side" (Fletcher 2011).

Alternatively, there are market segments where evidence suggests that higher-quality and therefore more costly ingredients can be profitable. For example, the fastest-growing segment in the dining area is called fast casual, which includes restaurants like Chipotle and Panera (Trefis 2014). *Fast casual restaurants* are known for using fresher, higher-quality, and more expensive inputs in their menus, but also fast service and a higher price point for menu items.[4] The typical price point for a fast casual restaurant falls in the $8 to $15 range, which falls between the quick service restaurant (e.g., Burger King) price point of less than $8 and the casual dining restaurant (e.g., Olive Garden) price point of at least $13 (Trefis 2014).

So what does this limited evidence tell us about the profitability of unhealthy foods relative to healthy foods? Nothing definitive, except that a categorical statement like "healthy foods *cannot* be profitable" is just as naïve and inaccurate as the categorical statement "healthy foods *can* be profitable." One must objectively consult the evidence on costs and revenues in the particular market (e.g., food item, location, time period). But surely there is a profitability framework that provides greater general insights and circumvents the pitfalls of categorical statements? Yes, there is: read on.

Most food companies sell more than one food item (e.g., a grocery store, a food processor, a fast food restaurant). A question they confront daily is this:

How many unhealthy products and how many healthy products should be produced in order to maximize profits?

To solidify and simplify the concepts, let's conceptually sort their mix of products on a continuous scale from healthy to unhealthy. There will be some optimal product mix of healthy and unhealthy foods that maximizes profit; any other mix will lead to a lower profit. This logic suggests a graph such as Figure 13.4, where the vertical axis denotes profit and the horizontal axis indicates the percentage of unhealthy foods being offered. The profit functions for two firms are shown.

Each point on a profit function corresponds to a specific profit level associated with a specific mix of unhealthy and healthy foods (e.g., 25% unhealthy, 75%

---

[4] Unfortunately, to muddy the water, higher-quality ingredients are not a sufficient condition for a healthier menu, as consumers can still eat unhealthy portion sizes of healthy foods. For example, Chipotle uses higher-quality ingredients, but the typical Chipotle order contains as many calories as its "unhealthy" competitors, if not more (Chandler 2015).

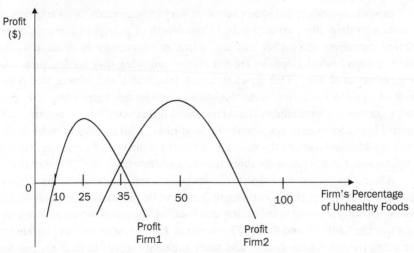

FIGURE 13.4 Two Firms' Profits with Respect to Percentage of Unhealthy Foods Offered.
[IAPS] Different firms have different mixes of healthy and unhealthy foods that serve different market segments and maximize their profits.

healthy). Note that prior to about 10% unhealthy foods, Firm 1 is losing money because its profit is negative.

Firm 1's profit function reaches a maximum by selling about 25% unhealthy foods and about 75% healthy foods; after that, profits decline as more unhealthy items are sold. Alternatively, Firm 2 maximizes its profit by selling about 50% healthy items and about 50% unhealthy items.

This graph is useful for multiple reasons. Note there is a range around 35% unhealthy items (65% healthy items) where both firms are making a positive profit, but neither is making the most it can. If Firm 1 increases the percentage of unhealthy items toward 50%, then its profit decreases and actually becomes negative. But also note that if Firm 2 tried to sell healthier items (move toward Firm 1's distribution), its profit would decrease as well. So what is going on here?

Figure 13.4 conveys one of the most fundamental concepts in economics and marketing: market segmentation. *Market segmentation* refers to the idea of dividing a large market into smaller segments of consumers or businesses with common preferences, demands, and capabilities. Market segmentation requires differences in consumers and/or firms and can occur along many dimensions (e.g., geographically, demographically, or just temporally). In the present context it simply means not everyone likes or produces the same food at the same time. A firm's ability to respond to market segments will be determined by its technological, managerial, and financial resources. Therefore, different firms will have different profit functions in different segments of the market, as shown in Figure 13.4.

So why can't all firms sell more healthy items? Market segmentation by definition means there are different markets of different sizes. Adam Smith's observation from Chapter 12 that the degree of specialization is limited by the extent of the market indicates that there is a limit to the degree to which firms can specialize in healthy or unhealthy foods and remain profitable. Figure 13.4 shows this graphically. The extent of the (profitable) market can be limited because either there are too few consumers in the market segment or the market segment is already crowded with many producers. For example, even though the fast casual market segment is growing, it still constitutes only 5% of all restaurant traffic (Ferdman 2015). But because it is the fastest-growing segment, it has gained the attention of firms in other segments trying to mimic its success.

Profit and Corporate Social Responsibility

As mentioned in Chapter 11, the media and academic and political circles are replete with strong criticisms and defenses of the role of the food industry in contributing to the "obesogenic food environment" (e.g., Bachus and Otten 2015; Desrochers and Shimizu 2012; Freedhoff 2014; Kraak et al. 2011; Lusk 2013; Moss 2014; Pollan 2006; Story, Hamm, and Wallinga 2009; Stuckler and Nestle 2012; Swinburn et al. 2015; Yach 2014). Many of these arguments, on both sides of the debate, come across as more hyperbole and subjective than balanced and objective and do not provide an analytical framework for analyzing the underlying incentives and their implications for the various stakeholders. This section extends the previous one and provides some tools for a more constructive dialogue.

Nutrition, public health, medical, and some policy stakeholders are calling on food firms ("Big Food") to be more socially responsible. Over the past 15 years CSR has become an increasingly important component of firms' decision making (Crook 2005). Not surprisingly, theoretical research on CSR has followed suit (e.g., Crifo and Forget 2015; Husted and Salazar 2006; Jensen 2002; McWilliams and Siegel 2001). Here we use the general definition of CSR given by McWilliams and Siegel (2001 p.117): "actions that appear to further some social good, beyond the interests of the firm and that which is required by law." Importantly, recognize that a firm that is simply placing nutrition facts on its food items or following food-safety regulations is not engaged in CSR but merely abiding by the law.

Given that firms are concerned about CSR, let's expand the firm's objective function (its utility) to include two components: profit and CSR. CSR is related to how much the firm is willing to invest in social goodwill capital. *Social goodwill capital* is any activity (e.g., changing its product mix, advertising, charity donations) that improves the company's public social image in aggregate (i.e., to the majority of individuals). To tie this to our earlier analysis, let social goodwill capital be measured by the percentage of unhealthy foods, G, produced by the firm. For some, the only level of G that maximizes CSR would be zero (i.e., no unhealthy food), but a more realistic value would be something greater than zero (e.g., $G = 35\%$). Regarding profit, as before, there will also be some optimal combination of unhealthy and healthy foods G that will maximize profits. Thus, in

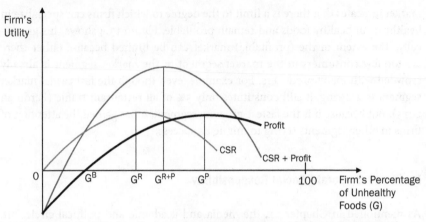

FIGURE 13.5 Firm's Utility from Corporate Social Responsibility and Profit with Percentage of Unhealthy Foods Placed on Market.

[IAPS] The firm's percentage of unhealthy foods will be determined by weighing the utility from corporate social responsibility versus profit.

choosing the level of G the firm must take into account the benefits (utility) it gets from both profits and the CSR.

Figure 13.5 gives a graphical representation of the tradeoff the firm is facing.[5] The curve labeled CSR represents the utility the firm receives from being socially responsible. This curve reflects the preferences of those who want the firm to be socially responsible. The firm's social responsibility would be maximized at G^R (e.g., 35% unhealthy). Greater than G^R and the social responsibility begins to decline. The curve labeled "profit" represents the utility for the firm associated with profits. Profit is positive and increasing between G^B and G^P. The mix of unhealthy and healthy foods that maximizes profit is G^P (e.g., 65% unhealthy). Now, because the firm receives utility from both the CSR and profit, it must integrate these into some common objective function. Here we just add them together, as shown by the curve CSR + profit. The value of G that maximizes the combined objective is G^{R+PR}, which is effectively a compromise between the two component optimal levels (e.g., 50% unhealthy). So the firm is *not* maximizing the CSR in isolation and it is also *not* maximizing profit in isolation, but it *is* maximizing their combination. Any move to the left of G^{R+PR} would increase CSR, but the decrease in profit would be greater. Any move to the right of G^{R+PR} would increase profit, but the decrease in CSR would be greater.

The above analysis reveals a fundamental point that must be grasped to make any headway on this issue: *The incentives for CSR maximization and profit maximization are incompatible over the relevant range of alternatives.* Over the relevant

---

[5] Figure 13.5 is a compromise graph and should look rather similar to the one found in Chapters 3 and 8, where the consumer was trading off hedonic utility with health utility. The same analytical concepts apply.

range of alternatives, as the CSR value increases, profits are decreasing, and vice versa. There is an inherent tension between the two objectives. One should also recognize the implications of a more fundamental distinction between the CSR and the profit objective: the units. The unit for profit is dollars, which is objective, tangible, and measurable and provides a very clear scorecard in terms of determining whether the firm is improving or declining. Alternatively, there is no objective, common, observable unit for CSR other than the satisfaction level (utility) of the special interest group, which is very subjective, even if quantifiable. Furthermore, because a firm comprises multiple individuals and the CSR units are subjective, even within the firm there are likely to be different opinions on the actual level of CSR the firm is achieving. Consequently, it is inherently difficult to merge these two objectives into one overall objective that will provide clear direction for management (Jensen 2002).

This of course leads to the natural question:

Are there circumstances where the incentives for profit maximization and CSR are compatible?

The general answer is yes, in the case of a *strategic CSR* (Husted and Salazar 2006). In the *strategic CSR* case, a firm's investment in CSR increases not only its CSR value but also its profitability. The incentive to increase profit is compatible with increasing CSR value and vice versa.[6] This in turn solves the units problem, because if CSR and profits are positively related, then the firm can be assured that increasing profits is also increasing the CSR. In this case, CSR is a "win–win" scenario. What would that look like graphically? The strategic CSR case amounts to shifting the location of the profit function such that it will be maximized at the same point where the CSR is maximized, and that is achieved by perhaps radically changing the business model.

Unfortunately, the "win–win" strategic CSR case is difficult to achieve on a grand scale because it is very hard to find win–win scenarios for both consumers and producers. On the consumer side, consumers generally want cheap, convenient food that tastes good, because they have other things they want to spend their money and time on besides food and good-tasting food is preferred to bad-tasting food. On the producer side, it is not enough that consumers say they like healthier food; they must be willing to pay for it, and the price premium must be greater than any increase in the cost. So the strategic CSR trick is to figure out ways to get consumers to pay a sufficient premium for healthier foods that will cover the additional cost *or* reduce the cost of consuming and producing healthier foods.

---

[6] Jensen (2002, p. 238) states the problem concisely: "It is logically impossible to maximize in more than one dimension at the same time unless the dimensions are monotone transformations of one another." Translation? The multiple objectives must be positively related so as the value of one increases (decreases), the value of the other increases (decreases) over all relevant ranges of the decision-making process. If this condition is not satisfied, then CSR acts as a constraint on profits, and it is easy to prove mathematically, using the Le Chatelier principle, that profits will *always* be lower by adding the CSR constraint.

Distributing the Profits and Goodwill

1. What implications do you think the concepts of market segmentation and specialization being limited by the extent of the market have for nutrition policies targeting unhealthy foods?

2. As we have discussed, many stakeholders in the food environment often take vehement and polemic positions regarding the food environment and the distribution of unhealthy foods in the food system. What would Figure 13.5 look like if CSR was maximized at zero (i.e., the optimal CSR value was $G = 0$)? Does this help explain why some advocacy groups may take extreme positions in the media? Explain. Repeat this exercise from the industry perspective where some may *claim* profit is maximized far to the right.

3. The idea of incentive compatibility is an important concept when confronting different objectives. Though taxing unhealthy foods and subsidizing healthy foods may be considered opposite sides of the same coin, discuss why one incentive is compatible with CSR and profit and the other is not.

Conclusions

The food marketing sector consists of millions of firms, but the same fundamental economic principles apply to all: the output decision still depends on how revenues *and* costs change as the output is changed. Revenue or cost changes in isolation are insufficient to indicate whether the change will be profitable; instead, *both* must be considered. The literature is filled with research suggesting that consumers will pay a premium for product Y with healthy attribute Z. But without considering the cost side as well, such findings tell us nothing about profitability and therefore financial sustainability.

Our food supply is heavily skewed toward high-fat, high-sugar, and high-sodium foods. This distribution reflects differences in consumers' preferences and demands and producers' capabilities and resources and thus market segmentation principles and limits. Perhaps not surprisingly, then, there is also a diverse set of opinions about working with the food industry to improve the food environment, ranging from a call to arms and confrontation (e.g., Koplan and Brownell 2010), to cooperation (e.g., Freedman 2014; Yach 2014), to suggesting cautious but skeptical dialogue (e.g., Freedhoff 2014; Stuckler and Nestle 2012). The framework on CSR presented here helps to cut through the rhetoric and provides a framework for understanding the issues and positions. Unless the incentives for CSR are compatible with the firm's objective (i.e., the strategic CSR case), the tension will remain between those interested in increasing CSR and firms looking to improve their financial standing. In this case neither side will be completely satisfied. The difficult trick is to find incentives that are compatible with both the CSR objective and the profit objective and that involve understanding the economics of revenue *and* cost, not just one or the other. As stated in the *Economist* (Crook 2005, p. 4), "To improve capitalism, you first need to understand it." Our understanding will deepen as we head to our next destination in the journey—the market, where consumers and producers come together.

Closing Conversation

JP: You weren't kidding. Between the concert and talking through this topic, it's 2:30 a.m.! But I learned two main things. First, the same general principles apply for a food company or a restaurant or even a beekeeper. The change in cost must be offset by a greater change in revenue in order for the change to be profitable. Second, there is a tension between the objectives of those interested in corporate social responsibility and *some* firms trying to maximize profits. Market segmentation and the limits of the market suggest that there will be some firms that can offer healthier foods, but not all. The best way to change the distribution of foods toward healthier foods is to figure out ways to make them more profitable.

Margaret: Yeah. Those are the basic points. I also see this as a great opportunity for you and your profession because as consumers demand healthier foods— recognizing in economic terms that demand means not just "like" but also "willing to pay"—food companies will have to respond.

JP: We have an obvious respect for each other's work. I like that.

PART IV

The Determination of Food Prices and Quantities in Competitive Markets

This section of the book covers the determination of food prices and quantities in competitive markets. Chapter 14 addresses the question: Who determines the prices and quantities of food in our food system? Consumers? Producers? Both? We demonstrate and discuss why market prices and quantities occur where market supply and demand curves intersect. We show how changes in demand and supply will affect prices and quantities in the market. Chapter 15 demonstrates how markets may be related either horizontally or vertically. We show how changes in demand and supply in one market will affect prices and quantities in another market. In both chapters, we analyze recent topics related to food and nutrition policy, such as a sugar-sweetened beverage tax and corn subsidies.

PART IV

The Determination of Food Prices and Quantities in Competitive Markets

14

Demand and Supply
PRICES AND QUANTITIES IN A COMPETITIVE MARKET

Learning Objectives

What you will know by the end of this chapter:

- ¤ the definitions of consumer sovereignty and producer sovereignty;
- ¤ the definition of a market;
- ¤ the role of prices in a market;
- ¤ how market equilibrium price and quantity are determined using a supply and demand framework;
- ¤ how effective a food or beverage tax will be in reducing caloric intake and how much of the tax will be paid by consumers; and
- ¤ what happens to market price and quantity if multiple factors are changing.

Opening Conversation

JP [walking his dog with Margaret]: Something doesn't make sense in this economic framework. At first you told me that consumers are responding to predetermined prices. Then you told me that producers are responding to predetermined prices, except in that case where producers set prices. Well, who determines prices if it is not producers? I mean, it seems to me that the consumer is at the mercy of the firms that sell food products. However, I realize that by competition firms cannot do anything they want. So I guess the ultimate question is this: How are market prices and quantities determined?

Margaret: I really enjoy talking to you about this stuff, because it is so obvious that you think deeply about this stuff and really want to understand it. Let me see if I can explain it.

Who Determines Prices and Quantities: Consumers? Producers? Or Both?

Sections II and III of the book presented the economics of consumer demand and producer supply based on predetermined prices, respectively, except in the price-making producer section of Chapter 13. But who determines prices and therefore quantities? Producers? Consumers? Or both?

One of the oldest debates in economics is that of consumer sovereignty versus producer sovereignty (see Persky 1993 for a history). *Consumer sovereignty* is the assertion that consumers' choices determine firms' production choices. Producers are just responding to the desires of consumers in the goods they produce. Consumers are king. Consumption drives production. Demand determines supply. In contrast, *producer sovereignty* is the assertion that firms' choices determine consumers' choices. Firms create goods and use marketing techniques to sell consumers the goods that the firm wants to sell, not necessarily the goods consumers want to buy. Consumers are just responding to producers. Producers are king. Production drives consumption. Supply determines demand.

The criticisms and defenses of "Big Food" being responsible for our current food environment are really just debates about consumer versus producer sovereignty, though those terms are never used. Critics and consumer advocacy groups tend to be producer sovereigntists. Defenders and producer advocacy groups tend to be consumer sovereigntists. Which view is correct? As with most extreme views, the truth lies somewhere in the middle. As long as a consumer or producer has some freedom to participate or not in the market, then complete consumer or producer sovereignty will not exist. Rather, the difference between consumer sovereignty and producer sovereignty is more a matter of degree of market power. The degree of consumer or producer market power will vary by the specific good, market, time, and location. In his brilliant scissors analogy, Alfred Marshall, one of the fathers of economics, states it this way:

> We might as reasonably dispute whether it is the upper or the under blade of a pair of scissors that cuts a piece of paper, as whether value is governed by utility [demand] or cost of production [supply]. It is true that when one blade is held still and the cutting is effected by moving the other, we may say with careless brevity that the cutting is done by the second; but the statement is not strictly accurate, and is to be excused only so long as it claims to be merely a popular and not a strictly scientific account of what happens. (Marshall, 1920, p. 348)

So how do the blades of the scissors of supply and demand come together to determine prices and quantities?

Market Prices and Quantities: What Does a Plot Show?

Recall that the demand curve shows that as price decreases, quantity demanded increases, *ceteris paribus*. The supply curve shows that as price increases, quantity supplied increases, *ceteris paribus*. Now look at Figure 14.1, which gives a plot of annual prices and quantities for fresh potatoes in the United States from 2007 to

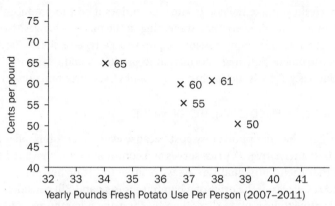

FIGURE 14.1 Annual Market Prices and Quantities of Fresh Potatoes in the United States, 2007-2011.

Source: Data from U.S. Department of Agriculture, National Agricultural Statistics Service 2011.

2011. What do you see? As the price decreases more is consumed, so these must be points on a demand curve, right? That seems correct when the price is 65, 55, and 50 cents, but not when the price is 60 and 61 cents. The quantity consumed at the higher price of 60 cents is the same as when the price is 55 cents. Furthermore, when the price increases to 61 cents, consumption increases. Perhaps these two points show a supply curve, because as the price increases the quantity increases? No, that is inconsistent with the first three points. No, something else is going on.

Defining a Market and the Important Role of Prices

Let's start from the beginning. Prices and quantities are determined within markets. But what is a market? A *market* is a collection of individuals or entities buying and selling a good or goods, where the term "good" generally includes services. The individuals or goods do not have to be in spatial or even temporal proximity. Exporters in Brussels and importers in the United States buy and sell goods (e.g., Brussels sprouts?) without being in the same spatial location. Individuals buy and sell insurance every day (e.g., protection against future events, like a flood). The key element of a market is that it is a system for allocating resources between consumers and producers (i.e., buyers and sellers). Consumers are allocating their resources (e.g., money, time, knowledge) to purchase goods they desire to increase utility, broadly defined. Producers are allocating their resources (e.g., money, time, skills) to sell goods to satisfy some objective, usually maximizing profit. Very simply stated, producers have something consumers want and consumers have something producers want.

So if markets are about solving a resource allocation problem between consumers and producers, this requires an exchange of information between consumers and producers revealing how they value the resources in question. What should the instrument be for exchanging this information? A survey? What should the survey ask? What would you like to buy? What would you like to sell? On a scale of 1 to

5 how much do you like the good? How much does it cost to produce the good? Do we do a new survey every time something in the market changes? No, making the transaction as efficient as possible requires some type of simple, flexible, and dynamic instrument signaling information to producers and consumers concisely and continuously. Price is such an instrument and serves three functions in markets.

PRICES ACT AS A FIXED STANDARD OF VALUE

Every decision has an opportunity cost because every decision implies forgoing the next best alternative.[1] A price serves as a common unit with a fixed standard of value that each individual can assess relative to his or her personal preferences and resources. If the price of a hamburger is $4 and Bill considers the next best alternative to be a pizza slice, then by choosing a hamburger Bill gives up $4 worth of a pizza for eating the hamburger. Alternatively, if Ted considers the next best alternative to be a burrito, then Ted gives up $4 worth of a burrito for eating the hamburger. Therefore, the single price provides a fixed standard for comparing the worth or value of different goods to consumers and producers.

PRICES PROVIDE A SIGNAL FOR RESOURCE ALLOCATION

How do all the producers in an economy know which goods to produce and the consumers which goods to consume? The answer is prices. Because prices reflect value, they provide a signal to producers *and* consumers for guiding the organization of production- and consumption-related resources. For example, if a farmer can grow either tomatoes or strawberries and the price of strawberries is expected to be higher at harvest, then, assuming the cost of growing both is the same, the farmer would likely plant strawberries.

PRICES DETERMINE THE DISTRIBUTION
OF PRODUCTION AMONG CONSUMERS

Once a given amount of a good is produced, prices determine how production will be distributed among consumers. As the price of a good increases, it requires more of the consumer's income, and different people have different income levels. Alternatively viewed, more people can buy low-priced goods than high-priced goods, so prices serve an automatic distribution or rationing function in society.

In summary, the price mechanism also allows each party to individually determine how he or she would like to allocate his or her own resources without anyone dictating how to allocate them. A price preserves freedom of choice subject to personal resource constraints. Prices are the heart of a market system and serve as an extraordinarily simple yet sophisticated and sustainable way of providing information about the value of resources. Using Adam Smith's well-known metaphor, prices are the "invisible hand" that guides the allocation of resources in a market economy.

---

[1] This does not mean the next best alternative is desirable (e.g., a Hobsonian or dilemma type of choice).

Pause to Contemplate Alternative Food Systems

Given the definition of a market and the important role prices provide in a self-sustaining incentive environment for resource allocation, suppose you are dissatisfied with the local food system in your community and feel something needs to be done to improve the nutrition quality of foods being sold and consumed in the market. Propose two solutions and then evaluate them based on the following questions.

1. How has your solution changed incentives for the consumer given what you know about consumer constraints, substitutes, and opportunity cost? Explain.
2. How has your solution changed incentives for the producer given what you know about producer constraints, competition, opportunity cost, and profitability? Explain.
3. Is the system self-sustaining? That is, what self-sustaining mechanisms exist in your food system for helping consumers *and* producers decide how to allocate resources toward more healthy foods? Explain.

Market Equilibrium in a Perfectly Competitive Market

Markets can be categorized by the level of competition. There are generally two categories: perfectly competitive markets and imperfectly competitive markets. This book covers only the perfectly competitive case. The perfectly competitive case is the most accessible to those without an economics background, and it is the foundation for comparison with imperfectly competitive models.[2] A *perfectly competitive market* is defined by the following conditions:

1. No single firm can affect the price in the market by changing its production.
2. No single consumer can affect the price in the market by changing his or her consumption.
3. There is perfect information available about prices and the good.
4. There is freedom of entry and exit from the market.
5. The good is homogeneous.

These may seem like extreme conditions to be satisfied in some markets. However, for most of the food sector, such as farms, wholesale food markets, and grocery stores, they are a very good approximation. For example, in the United States, when a farmer takes his corn to a grain elevator, he must accept the posted cash price for that day. Or again in the United States, when you go to the grocery store, you must pay the price posted. These assumptions may seem more debatable in

---

[2] This book is designed to be an introduction to the economics of food and nutrition. Models of imperfectly competitive markets, such as monopoly, duopoly, and oligopoly, are more advanced topics and can be found in most intermediate-level microeconomic textbooks, such as Varian (2006).

the food service sector (e.g., restaurants) but we covered that case in Chapter 13, so the reader can refer back to that analysis. However, even in the food service sector, the perfectly competitive model is still a good starting point as it will often provide many of the same directional (qualitative) insights that would be achieved with a more complicated imperfectly competitive model.

The *market demand curve* is just the sum of all individual consumer demand curves. The *market supply curve* is just the sum of all individual producer supply curves. Each point on a market demand and supply curve represents a market quantity demanded and supplied, respectively. The *market quantity equilibrium* is where the market quantity demanded equals the market quantity supplied (the curves intersect). The *market equilibrium price* is the price where the market quantity equilibrium occurs ("the market clears").

Figure 14.2 gives a graphical representation of the market equilibrium. The market supply and demand curves are represented by S and D, respectively. The market equilibrium price and quantity are represented by p_E and F_E, respectively. *All* quantities between 0 and F_E sell for and are bought at the same market equilibrium price, p_E. Why is this an equilibrium? Well, consider any other price, such as p_0, and note what will happen. At p_0 the quantity demanded, F_1, is greater than the quantity supplied, F_0, so there is a *shortage* in the market. Remember, by the definition of the demand curve, at the quantity F_0 some consumers would be willing to pay a maximum of p_1 for this quantity. Consequently, consumers will start to compete with each other by offering higher prices for the fixed amount of F_0. As the offer price starts to rise, two things happen. First, some individuals drop out or demand less, and because the price is going up, producers will begin to produce more. Thus, as the price is bid up, the quantity demanded is decreasing and the quantity supplied is increasing, and this process continues until p_E and F_E are reached.

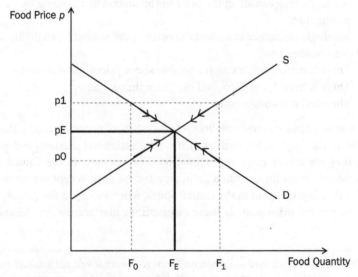

FIGURE 14.2 Market Equilibrium Price and Quantity.
[IAPS] The market clearing price and quantity occurs where supply equals demand.

Why does this process not continue past p_E? Well, suppose it did, such as at p_1. Now the reverse process occurs. At price p_1 there is now a *surplus* because the quantity supplied, F_1, is greater than the quantity demanded, F_0. Given this excess supply, producers will not be able to sell everything they have brought to the market at this price, so in order to keep from just throwing away the excess supply and not get anything for it, they will start to compete with each other by offering a lower price in order to sell the excess. As this occurs, the quantity demanded increases, but the decreasing price leads to a decrease in the amount brought to the market, so the quantity supplied is decreasing. This process continues until the market equilibrium point is reached. It should be clear from this description that it takes two to tango: consumers and producers. Neither is sovereign when it comes to determining the market price and quantity.[3]

Changes in Market Equilibrium

The market equilibrium prices and quantities will change as demand and supply shift. Remember, a shift in a curve occurs because some variable affecting demand or supply *other than the price of the good* has changed. We covered individual demand shifters in Chapters 3 through 10 and individual supply shifters in Chapters 12 and 13, and all of those apply here at the market level. At the market level we also need to add the number of consumers for demand and the number of producers for supply as shifters as well. This should make sense. The more consumers, *ceteris paribus*, the more demand. The more producers, *ceteris paribus*, the more supply. Table 14.1 gives a summary of the different market demand and supply shifters.

Figure 14.3 shows what will happen to the market price and quantity as market demand shifts out *or* supply shifts out. As demand shifts out (panel A) the price and quantity in the market are expected to increase.

Alternatively, as supply shifts out (panel B) the price is expected to decrease but the quantity is expected to increase. The graph in panel A would be consistent with any of the shifters given in Column 2 of Table 14.1. For example, in the market for vegetables, we would expect an increase in income, or an increase in available time, or an increase in the cooking skills via cooking education information to all increase demand. The graph in panel B would be consistent with any of the shifters given in Column 3 of Table 14.1. In the vegetable market, this would be factors such as a decrease in the price of an input, such as labor, or an increase in the number of vegetable producers, and so forth. Note that all of these results are symmetrical in that the market demand and supply curves would shift in if these variables moved in the opposite direction from that given in Table 14.1.

---

[3] In anticipation of the complaint that the assumptions of perfect competition rule out consumer or producer sovereignty by definition, we would respond thusly. Even in the extreme cases of monopoly and monopsony, complete producer or consumer sovereignty will not occur. Monopoly does not mean the consumer must buy the product, only that there is only one firm that sells it. Consequently, the monopolist is still limited by the extent of the market as represented by the demand curve. On the monopsony side (only one buyer), similar logic applies, as the single buyer must still interact with multiple sellers and is influenced by their desires and capabilities.

TABLE 14.1

Effects of Different Variables on Market Demand and Supply Curves

General Curve Effect	Market Demand Curve	Market Supply Curve
Movement down along curve *if*	*Own price p decreases ↓*	*Own price p decreases ↓*
Movement up along curve *if*	*Own price p increases ↑*	*Own price p increases ↑*
Shift **out** →[a] *if*	*Own time cost-related variables, w or t, decrease ↓*	*Substitute price in production p^s decreases ↓*
	Substitute price in consumption p^s increases ↑	*Complement price p_c in production increases ↑*
	Substitute time cost-related variables, w_s or t_s, increase ↑	*Normal input price r decreases ↓*
	Complement price in consumption p_c decreases ↓	*Technology G increases ↑*
	Complement time cost-related variables, w_c or t_c, decrease ↓	*Number of producers K increase ↑*
	Cognitive processing cost e decreases ↓	
	Behavioral effect variables that increase demand ↑	
	Money budget M increases ↑ (for normal good)	
	Time budget T increases ↑ (for normal good)	
	Enhancing information I increases ↑	
	Number of consumers N increase ↑	

[a] Curves would "shift in" if variables moved in the opposite directions from those given in the table.

At this point you should realize what was going on in the plot of potato prices and quantities (see Fig. 14.1). Each point represents an intersection of market supply and demand. Note that each point is indicated by a × mark, like a little supply and demand intersection. An accidental marker choice? Not! A change in a point means that one of three things happened: (1) some other demand factor (e.g., income) caused the demand to shift and supply stayed constant, (2) some other supply factor (e.g., weather) caused supply to shift and demand stayed constant, or (3) demand and supply both shifted. Stated more succinctly, points on a scatter plot do *not* hold other factors constant.

THE INCIDENCE OF THE TAX AND CHANGES IN CONSUMPTION AND CALORIES

The actual magnitude of the shifts in Figure 14.3 will vary depending on the variable that is changing, the magnitude of the change, and the slopes of the demand and the

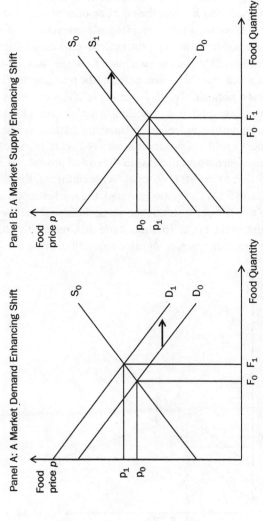

FIGURE 14.3 A Market Change Induced by a Single Demand *or* Supply Shift.

[IAPS] Price and quantity move in the same direction when market demand shifts. Price and quantity move in opposite directions when market supply shifts.

supply curves. A classic case of where the slope of the market demand and supply curve is very important is what is known as the incidence of the tax. As we discussed in Chapter 5, a sugar-sweetened beverage tax has been discussed as a way to reduce caloric intake. Suppose that the price per ounce of a sugar-sweetened beverage is about 6.25 cents, or about $1 for a 16-ounce drink. Furthermore, suppose the proposed tax is 2 cents per ounce sold, a 32% tax rate. There are two obvious questions of interest: (1) How effective will such a tax be in decreasing caloric intake? (2) How much of this tax will be passed on to the consumer? The typical answer you see in the media is "it will be very effective because the entire amount of the tax will be passed on to the consumer." Let's see what the economic analysis reveals about this answer.

First, note that each ounce of a food product will have a constant number of calories. For example, an ounce of Coca-Cola has about 12 calories. To apply this concept to any food, let's define a calorie conversion factor c. The total calories C in a food is then determined by the equation $C = c \times F$. For example, if $F_0 = 1,000$ and $c = 12$, then $C_0 = 12,000$. Consequently, as this is just a rescaling of the horizontal food axis, we can just draw another horizontal line under the food quantity axis that represents calories.

Now, for every ounce sold, the producer must pay 2 cents, or more generally τ. The 2 cents, or τ, is equivalent to an increase in the cost of production, so the market supply curve will shift to the left (Fig. 14.4). Without the tax, the initial market equilibrium tax is p_0 and F_0. With the tax imposed, the market supply curve shifts from S_0 to S_1. Given this is a per unit tax, the vertical distance between S_0 and S_1 is equal to the amount of the tax τ. To understand this, remember that the price on the supply curve equals the *minimum* price required to bring the good to the

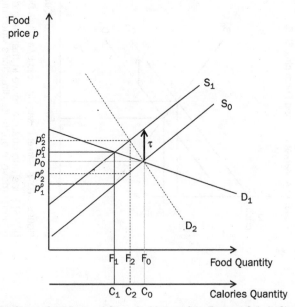

FIGURE 14.4 The Slope of the Demand Curve, Incidence of the Tax, and Calorie Change.
[IAPS] The steeper the demand curve (i.e., the more inelastic), the larger the price increase, the smaller the quantity decrease, and the smaller the calorie decrease. The more inelastic the demand curve, the larger the proportion of the tax paid by the consumer and the smaller the portion paid by the producer.

market. If producers must pay the tax, then they are going to have to receive $p_0 + \tau$ to supply the same quantity as before the tax because once they pay the tax, then they would receive the same initial price p_0 (i.e., $p_0 = (p_0 + \tau) - \tau$). With the tax, the new equilibrium would occur at the quantity F_1 and the new calorie level would be C_1. At this quantity, the new price the consumer faces is read off the demand curve and is p_1^c. However, because the producers must pay the tax τ, they receive what the consumers pay *less* the tax or $p_1^p = p_1^c - \tau$, the "effective price." Because the per unit tax is the vertical distance between the two supply curves, we can just read the price the producers receive off the lower supply curve S_0. The tax acts as a wedge between the price the consumers pay and the price the producers receive. The amount of the tax is therefore shared by the consumers and the producers in that the consumers pay $p_1^c - p_0$ of the tax and the producers pay $p_0 - p_1^p$ such that when we sum the amount paid by each we get the tax, $\tau = (p_1^c - p_0) + (p_0 - p_1^p)$.

Now consider the role of the elasticity (slope) of the demand curve. If the demand curve were more inelastic, as represented by the dotted curve D_2, the tax would cause a greater price increase (p_0 to p_2^c) relative to the quantity decrease (F_0 to F_2) and the decrease in caloric intake is not as great (C_0 to C_2) as when demand is more elastic. Note also that consumers are now paying more of the tax and producers are paying less. How the tax is distributed between consumers and producers is known as the *incidence of the tax*. The incidence of the tax is determined by the elasticities (slopes) of the demand and supply curves.

Master Manipulator

To check your understanding of market equilibrium determination, work through these questions:

1. Think of two very specific foods. Think of two very specific causes for demand to *shift in* for these two foods (hint: use Table 14.1) and show these on a graph. Discuss what happens to the market equilibrium price and quantity.
2. Repeat #1 for supply.
3. As indicated, we often hear someone say, "The tax will be passed on fully to the consumer." What does this statement implicitly assume about the demand or supply elasticities (slopes)? Is there a case where producers pay the full amount of the tax? Show and explain both cases graphically (hint: use Fig. 14.4 and think extremes).

MULTIPLE SHIFTS IN MARKET DEMAND OR SUPPLY CURVES

We have only considered a single shift in one curve in the market. However, there can be multiple factors changing that lead to multiple shifts in market demand or supply. For example, the demand for vegetables may increase if income increases, but the supply of vegetables may decrease if harvesting costs increase. Analytically, just proceed by taking one shift at a time and add them together.

Figure 14.5 gives two rather general cases: (A) when demand and supply shift in the same direction and (B) when demand and supply shift in opposite directions. In

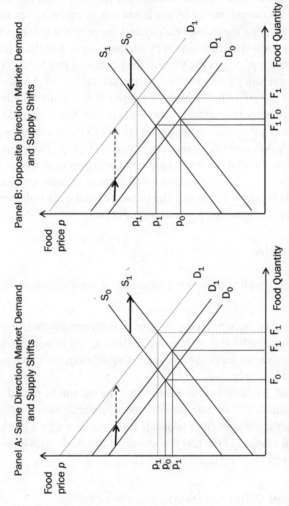

Panel A: Same Direction Market Demand
and Supply Shifts

Panel B: Opposite Direction Market Demand
and Supply Shift

FIGURE 14.5 A Market Change Induced by a Market Demand and Supply Shift.

[IAPS] When demand and supply shift in the same direction, qualitative quantity effects can
be determined but not price effects. When demand and supply shift in opposite directions,
qualitative price effects can be determined but not quantity effects.

panel A something has caused demand for the food to *increase* (e.g., a health education program) but something has also caused the supply of the food to *increase* (e.g., an increase in the number of sellers). Both shifts are reinforcing the positive quantity effect, but the increase in demand increases price and the increase in supply decreases price. Whether the price will increase or decrease depends on the size of the relative shifts. For example, the solid demand curve D_1 shows a small demand shift relative to the supply shift, so the price decreases in this case to the dark p_1. However, if the increase in demand was greater, as shown by the dotted demand D_1, then the price of the food would increase to the lighter p_1. Note the quantity, however, still increased.

In panel B something has caused demand for the food to *increase* (e.g., a decrease in the time cost) but something has also caused the supply of the food to *decrease* (e.g., an increase in a cost of production, such as a tax). In this case, while both shifts are reinforcing the price effect, they are offsetting with respect to quantity. Now whether quantity increases or decreases depends on the size of the individual shifts. For example, the solid demand curve D_1 shows a small demand shift relative to the supply shift, so the quantity decreases in this case to the dark F_1.

However, if the increase in demand was greater as shown by the dotted demand D_1, then the quantity of the food would increase to the lighter F_1. Figure 14.5 demonstrates a recurring theme: when there are multiple factors changing, then counterintuitive results can emerge if one considers only a single effect in isolation as an explanation.

Multiple Master Manipulator

Many nutrition policies are designed to offset other environmental factors. Most of these policies are targeted at consumers. Use your knowledge of multiple shifts to answer the following questions:

1. It is well documented that the number of fast food restaurants has increased over the past two decades. Using the list of variables in Table 14.1, identify which variables would be expected to change, and then draw the associated supply and demand diagram and the expected effect on caloric intake. Explain in words.
2. Given #1, use the list of variables in Table 14.1 to identify possible policy instruments the government could use to offset or moderate this supply environment effect. Show and explain your choice graphically.

Conclusions

In this chapter we have covered some of the most fundamental concepts in economics: the definition of a market, the role of prices, and supply and demand. Prices and quantities are determined where demand *and* supply interact. Changes in prices and quantities are the result of changes in demand *and* supply. The magnitude of these changes will depend on the elasticities (slopes) of the market demand and supply curves. We demonstrated the importance of these concepts in the context of a tax on sugar-sweetened beverages with the goal of reducing caloric intake. The effectiveness of such a policy in reducing caloric intake and how much of the tax will be passed on to the consumer will depend on the elasticities of demand *and* supply. We also demonstrated how multiple changes in demand and supply can lead to offsetting effects in prices or quantities. This analysis reiterates a theme throughout the book: counterintuitive results associated with a market policy or instrument do *not* mean the policy is not having the desired effect; rather, it may be moderated or offset by some other factor.

Most efforts to improve nutrition are directed at consumers and the demand side of the market. Policy designs will be much more effective when they are evaluated in the context of the more comprehensive framework of a market (supply and demand), rather than assuming, to paraphrase Marshall, that only the demand blade of the scissors determines prices, quantities, and consequently nutrient intake and health. For example, in their award-winning article, Dharmasena, Davis, and Capps (2014) find that the effectiveness of a sugar-sweetened beverage tax is much more sensitive to assumptions about how producers respond—the supply side—than how consumers respond—the demand side. Ignoring the supply side leads to an overestimation of the effectiveness of a sugar-sweetened beverage tax on consumption and caloric intake. We are well on our way in the journey to understand how markets operate. Now we need to go deeper to understand how markets are related, so let the journey continue.

Closing Conversation

JP: Ah, so that's how supply and demand works! I've always heard about the interaction of supply and demand but never knew exactly what that meant. So effectively, competition on both sides of the market determines market prices and quantities and will prevent complete consumer or producer sovereignty. Life is much simpler when you just blame consumers for making bad choices or producers for selling foods consumers don't really want. I'd like to consider under what conditions the soft drink tax would be passed on completely to the consumer. If I look at Figure 14.4 and the vertical distance between the supply curves is the amount of the tax, then in order for the consumer price to increase that full amount, the market supply curve would have to be a horizontal line—what you call perfectly elastic supply. Furthermore, if the market supply curve were perfectly elastic, then because the price to the consumer would increase a lot more, the consumption of soft drinks would decrease a lot more and the soft drink tax would be much more effective, correct? So the effectiveness of the tax really does depend on the slope of the supply curve as well.

Margaret: JP, that's exactly right. In fact, as I mentioned, that's one of the things that Dharmasena, Davis, and Capps found: that assumptions about the supply side of the market (i.e., about the supply elasticity) were more important than various assumptions on the demand side in terms of the effectiveness of a sugar-sweetened beverage tax.

JP: So I guess the moral is, it takes producers and consumers interacting to determine prices and quantities: "It takes two to tango," as they say.

Margaret: Yes, it does take two to tango. Do you like to dance?

15

Horizontally and Vertically Related Competitive Markets

Learning Objectives

What you will know by the end of this chapter:

- the difference between horizontally and vertically related markets;
- how to analyze horizontally and vertically related markets; and
- why ignoring market relationships can lead to over- or underestimating the impact of different nutrition policies.

Opening Conversation

JP [On the phone with Margaret]: Margaret, I had trouble sleeping last night because of you! I was thinking about the tango and I was thinking about markets and supply and demand. Your analysis is either (1) flawed, (2) internally inconsistent, or (3) incomplete. That is, back when we were talking about consumers' choices and demand, if the price of a substitute food increased, then the demand for the food you were focused on would increase. In the supply and demand analysis, this means two markets are related. What happens in one market will affect another market. Consider another case. When we were talking about supply beyond the farm gate, you said that if the price of an input increased, then the supply of the outputs would decrease. Now as you explained, the input market is also called the upstream market and the output market is often called the downstream market. Consequently, again, what happens in one market will affect another market. But your supply and demand analysis didn't take that into account. What do you say to that?

Margaret: I say you are one smart cookie and you are right. What you have just described are called horizontally and vertically related markets. Supply and demand analysis is certainly general enough to account for these observations. Here's how it would work.

Introduction

Last week you bought a chuck roast for dinner because the price of pork chops was too high. This week you notice that the price of a chuck roast has gone up. With a little economics under your belt, you wonder: Did the higher price of pork chops increase the demand for chuck roast and therefore lead to an increase in the price of chuck roast? Your curiosity continues: More generally, how are the prices of pork chops and chuck roast related at the national level over time? Figure 15.1 shows the monthly retail prices (indices) of pork chops and chuck roast for the United States from 2010 to 2015. They both have similar patterns up until the latter part of 2012, where the chuck roast price jumped and continued to increase but the pork chop price actually decreased. However, around the early part of 2013 they returned to having similar patterns. So while the prices seem to be related, they are not perfectly related.

What would cause the price of pork chops or the price of chuck roasts to behave this way? Given chuck roasts come from cattle and pork chops from hogs, and corn is a major source of feed for both, perhaps the price of corn and therefore the price of cattle (and hogs) changed, leading to a change in the price of chuck roast and pork chops. Figure 15.2 shows the same consumer chuck roast price in the top panel, a middle panel with the price of cattle, and then the bottom panel with the price of corn. Note that the chuck roast and cattle prices track rather closely (i.e., increase and decrease together) but not in perfect unison. What about cattle prices and corn prices? Comparing the cattle price to the corn price indicates a much more complicated relationship. Speaking rather broadly, both prices are increasing up until about the middle of 2013, but then they actually move in opposite directions. Similarly to Figure 15.1, there are times when the prices seem to move in the same direction but other times when they are moving in opposite directions. So corn prices are not perfectly related with cattle prices or the chuck roast or pork price. So is there a general reason why sometimes related markets move together and other times they do not?

These are two examples of interrelated markets; what happens in one market affects what happens in another market. Understanding the economics of interrelated

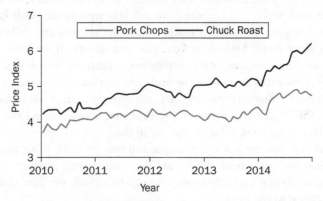

FIGURE 15.1 Monthly Consumer Price Indices for Pork Chops and Chuck Roast in the United States, 2010–2015.

Source: Bureau of Labor Statistics, Inflation and Prices 2015.

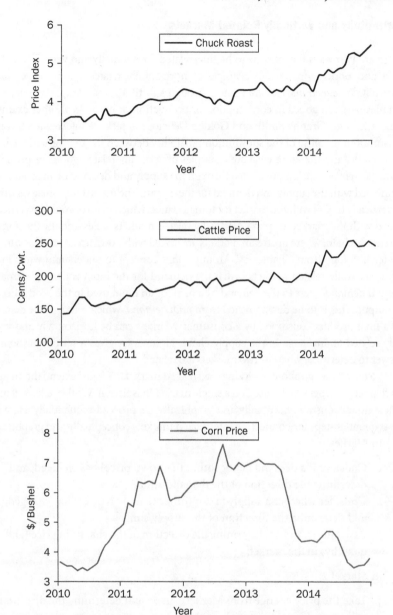

FIGURE 15.2 Consumer Price Index for Chuck Roast, Cattle Price, and Farm Corn Price in the United States, 2010–2015.

Source: Bureau of Labor Statistics, Inflation and Prices 2015, and U.S. Department of Agriculture, Economic Research Service, Feed Grains Yearbook 2015.

markets is extremely important when analyzing the impact of food policies or market interventions for two reasons. First, a well-intended policy targeted at one market can have unintended consequences in another untargeted market. Second, if we ignore the relationships between markets we likely will either over- or underestimate the change in prices and consumption associated with some policy or intervention. In this chapter we extend the supply and demand analysis in Chapter 14 to cover interrelated markets.

Horizontally and Vertically Related Markets

There are two ways for markets to be interrelated: horizontally and vertically. Chuck roast and pork chops are an example of horizontally related goods or products. *Horizontally related markets* are related through substitution or complementary possibilities between goods in consumption or production or both. As another example, the markets for Granny Smith and Golden Delicious apples are interrelated through consumption because of the substitution possibility between the two varieties. Chuck roast, cattle, and therefore corn are examples of vertically related goods or products. *Vertically related markets* are related through the supply and demand of an input being connected with the supply and demand for the output. The market for tomatoes would be vertically linked with the market for tomato sauce, which in turn would be vertically linked with the market for pizza. Vertically related markets are essentially the links in the supply chain, where upstream markets are linked with downstream markets, to use the terminology from Chapter 13. An important concept to understand when looking at vertically related markets is that the demand for the input is derived demand. *Derived demand* refers to the demand by a firm for an input used in the production of an output. This is to be distinguished from *final demand*, which refers to the demand for a final product consumed by a consumer. Markets can be horizontally and vertically related at any stage in the supply chain. Figure 15.3 gives a set of questions to answer to determine whether two markets are related.

So how do we go about analyzing interrelated markets? We just extend the analysis in Chapter 14, where we focused on a single market in isolation. While we look at markets simultaneously, conceptually and graphically we proceed sequentially. Here are the sequential steps for connecting interrelated markets conceptually and graphically.

In Market 1:

1. Consider if a demand factor (other than own price) has changed, and determine the direction of the demand shift.
2. Consider whether a supply factor (other than own price) has changed, and determine the direction of the supply shift.
3. Based on #1 and #2, determine the direction of the change in price (and quantity) in the market.

In Market 2:

4. Take the price change from Market 1 in #3 and determine the direction it will cause demand or supply to shift.
5. Shift the demand or supply accordingly.
6. Note the change in the market equilibrium price and quantity.

Notice that prices are the mechanisms that link markets. The price in one market affects the price in another market. Let's do a few examples.

The Analytics of Horizontally Related Markets

Let pork chops be Food 1 and chuck roast be Food 2. At the market level these foods are consumption substitutes. Suppose due to renegotiations of labor contracts, the

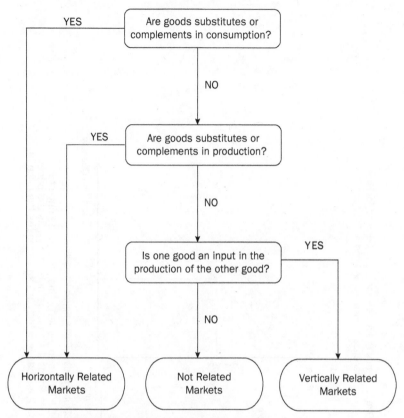

FIGURE 15.3 Flow Diagram for Determining Market Relationships.

hourly wage rate at hog processing plants increases. This is an increase in an input price (r_1). Panel A of Figure 15.4 shows what will happen in the market for pork chops (Food 1). The increase in the input price causes the supply curve to shift to the left (a decrease in supply). As the supply decreases, the price in the market increases from P_1^0 to P_1^1 and the equilibrium quantity in the market decreases from F_1^0 to F_1^1. None of this is new: this is exactly the type of analysis we did in Chapter 14.

The extension is to recognize that the increase in the price of pork chops (Food 1) may affect the demand for chuck roast (Food 2). Panel B shows the market for chuck roast (Food 2). As the price of pork chops increases (panel A), the demand for chuck roast (Food 2) would increase because the price of a substitute (pork chops) P_1 has increased. As the demand for chuck roast increases, the price and the quantity in the market increase from P_2^0 to P_2^1 and F_2^0 to F_2^1, respectively. Thus, the increase in the wage rate in the hog processing plants led to an increase in the price of pork chops and chuck roasts, as indicated in the introduction example. Note, however, the quantity of pork chops (Food 1) decreased and the quantity of chuck roasts (Food 2) increased. So for this case, the prices moved in the same direction but the quantities moved in opposite directions.

Let's consider another example where Figure 15.4 would apply. A recurring example throughout the book is a proposed tax on sugar-sweetened beverages (SSBs). In Chapter 14 we investigated the effects this would have on SSB consumption.

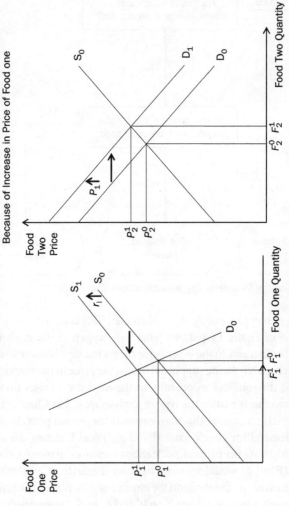
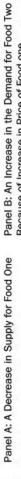

Panel A: A Decrease in Supply for Food One

Panel B: An Increase in the Demand for Food Two Because of Increase in Price of Food one

FIGURE 15.4 Horizontally Related Markets: Substitute Foods in Consumption Interacting.

[IAPS] As the supply decreases in Market 1 (shifts to the left), this causes the price to increase and quantity to decrease. Because Foods 1 and 2 are substitutes, as the price of Food 1 increases, the demand for Food 2 increases, which in turn increases the price of Food 2.

However, we did not consider what unintended consequences this may have on the consumption of other beverages, such as diet soft drinks, milk (high- and low-fat), or fruit juices. At the market level these other beverages would be considered substitutes for SSBs, so we would expect an SSB tax to have a "cross-price" effect and increase the demand for these other beverages. Consequently, Figure 15.4 describes this situation as well where Food 1 represents SSBs and Food 2 represents any or all other substitute beverages. Most importantly, the effectiveness of the tax at reducing calories will be *overestimated* if we ignore this cross-price effect. Just looking at panel A indicates that the quantity of SSBs (Food 1) would decrease, and therefore total caloric intake would decrease. However, because the other beverages are substitutes for SSBs, then as the price of SSBs increased due to the tax, then the demand for non-SSBs would increase, as shown in panel B. Consequently, caloric intake from these drinks would increase, offsetting to some degree the effect of the tax in decreasing caloric intake. Thus, ignoring the cross-price effect tends to *overestimate* the effectiveness of the tax. This overestimation has been documented in several studies (Dharmasena and Capps 2012; Finkelstein et al. 2013; Lin et al. 2011; Zhen et al. 2014), although Dharmasena, Davis, and Capps (2014) find that taking into account the supply side of the market is more important than taking into account these cross-price demand effects.

Figure 15.4 is very useful for conceptualizing some more general observations about horizontally related markets. In horizontally related markets:

1. The demand and supply curves will not generally have the same elasticity (slope) values.
2. The price and quantity changes in both markets do not have to be in the same direction or of the same magnitude.
3. If two goods are substitutes or complements in consumption, then their demand curves will be affected by the same variables.
4. If two goods are substitutes or complements in production, then their supply curves will be affected by the same variables.
5. Feedback between markets is continual, leading to continual changes in equilibrium prices and quantities.[1]

We hope these few examples give you an appreciation for the great flexibility and power this framework has for understanding the relationships between different markets, as the list of possibilities is almost endless. Consequently, this framework can be used to help explain why for some period of time two foods that are considered substitutes may have prices that move in the same direction and then at other times the prices appear to move in opposite directions. It takes both blades of the scissors to determine price, and if the individual blades in both markets are moving in similar directions, then the prices will move in similar directions, but if they are moving in opposite directions, so too will the price.

---

[1] The astute reader may ask: Doesn't the increase in price of Food 2 feed back and cause an increase in the demand for Food 1, which leads to an increase in the price of Food 1, which in turn leads to an increase in the demand for Food 2, and so forth? Yes, but this feedback does not continue indefinitely as the system is stable and converges to its new equilibrium because it is an underdamped dynamical system. The supply and demand diagram just shows the movements from one stable equilibrium to another, so the oscillations are not shown, just the final equilibrium values.

The Analytics of Vertically Related Markets

Suppose you have walked through the flowchart in Figure 15.3 and determined that two markets are vertically related as the output from one market (e.g., corn) is an input into another market (e.g., cattle). How should you proceed to analyze the interactions between the markets? The same as for horizontally related markets: changes in one market are transferred into another market.

Figure 15.5 demonstrates the analytics of vertically related markets when the supply in the upstream market increases. The top panel in Figure 15.5 represents the upstream market (e.g., corn) and the supply has shifted out, perhaps due to exceptional weather or a subsidy to grow corn provided by the government, which is denoted as an increase in v. As the supply increases from S_0 to S_1, the price decreases from p_0 to p_1 and the quantity increases from y_0 to y_1. Now the output in the upstream market (e.g., corn) is an input in the downstream market (e.g.,

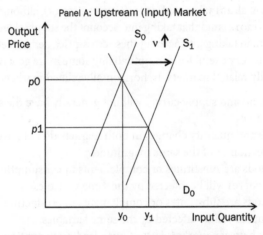

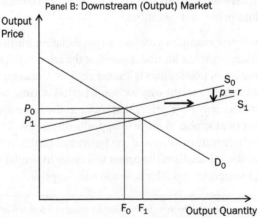

FIGURE 15.5 Vertically Related Markets: Input and Output Markets Interacting.

[IAPS] As the supply increases in the input market (shifts to the right), this causes the price to decrease and the quantity to increase (panel A). Because the input price has decreased, this causes the supply in the output market to increase and thus the price to decrease and the quantity to increase (panel B).

cattle). Thus the price of an input in the downstream market has decreased, and so the supply in the downstream market will increase from S_0 to S_1. This supply increase in turn leads to a decrease in the price in the downstream market (e.g., cattle) from P_0 to P_1 and an increase in the market quantity from F_0 to F_1.

Many of the general observations associated with horizontally related markets apply also for vertically related markets, but there are a few differences. In vertically related markets:

1. The output price and the quantity in the upstream market are the input price and the quantity in the downstream market.
2. The upstream derived demand curve will be affected by the same variables as the downstream supply curve.
3. The demand and supply curves in the upstream and downstream markets will not generally have to have the same elasticity (slope) values.
4. The price and quantity changes in the upstream and downstream markets do not have to be in the same direction or of the same magnitude.
5. feedback between markets is continual leading to continual changes in equilibrium prices and quantities.

Understanding the economics of vertically related markets is extremely important when evaluating the effects of interventions or policies in input markets on output markets and thus possible health. For example, a common claim is that corn subsidies in the United States have contributed to our obesity crisis (e.g., Huffpost 2013; Pianin 2012; Pollan 2003). The logic is that of vertically related markets. Corn subsidies make corn cheaper, which in turn makes high-fructose corn syrup cheaper, which in turn makes any food product that uses high-fructose corn syrup cheaper—thus, by the law of demand, consumers buy more foods with high-fructose corn syrup, which contributes to obesity, *ceteris paribus*. While the conceptual and directional logic is certainly sound, the conclusions are not, because of two caveats. First, as we have indicated above, the actual magnitudes of change are an empirical question depending on the demand and supply elasticities in all the markets. Second, there is the *ceteris paribus* caveat. Many other factors determine the prices and quantities in these markets. As we saw in Chapter 10, the actual share of the food dollar attributed to the food is usually less than 20%; in fact, Beghin and Jensen (2008) indicate that the farm value share in sweetened food is less than 5%. The most sophisticated analysis of the farm policy–obesity link has found very little empirical support for the argument that farm policies contribute much to the obesity crisis (e.g., Alston, Sumner, and Vosti 2008; Beghin and Jensen 2008; Okrent and Alston 2012; Rickard, Okrent, and Alston 2013; White 2008).

Questions of Connections

1. Construct a hypothetical story related to watermelon and cantaloupe where Figure 15.4 would apply.
2. How would the slope of the demand curve in Market 1 be related to the shift in the demand curve in Market 2? (Hint: Look at Fig. 15.4 and think extreme values.)
3. Use Figure 15.5 to help explain Figure 15.2 and the price relationships between chuck roast and cattle prices, but then also cattle price and corn. Given the

prices are not moving in perfect unison, construct a possible explanation using Figure 15.5 to explain how the prices may move in opposite directions.

Conclusions

In this chapter we extended the supply and demand analysis of single markets from Chapter 14 to the cases where markets are interrelated. There are two types of interrelationships: horizontal and vertical. Horizontally related markets occur when two markets (and their goods) are substitutes or complements in production or consumption. Vertically related markets occur when the output of one market is an input in another market. Understanding the economics of horizontally and vertically related markets is quite important, especially when evaluating the effects of different policies. Perhaps the most important point to come out of this chapter is that the effectiveness of policies will likely be overestimated (or underestimated) if one ignores the spillover effects of the policy into other markets. Thus, a complete policy analysis requires considering all markets that may be affected and for which there may be unintended consequences of the policy.

We are almost at the end of our journey, but there is one last stop. How do we determine if some intervention is cost-effective or if the benefits outweigh the cost? The last chapter will address this question.

Closing Conversation

JP: This is like playing with a Lego set: the possible connections seem endless! The horizontally related market example with the SSB tax really helped demonstrate how ignoring the effects on other markets can lead to an overstatement (or underestimate) of the effectiveness of a nutrition intervention or policy. This is a great example of the proverbial "unintended consequences." The explanation of the vertically related markets also makes sense as to why farm policies that subsidize corn production may not have as great an impact on food consumption, and therefore the obesity problem, as is often claimed in the popular press. I should have realized this result was likely once I recognized from our previous discussion that the percentage of actual raw product food cost in our foods is quite low. This economic framework is quite intricate but also quite useful for thinking about many different issues related to food and nutrition, but I can see it requires discipline of thought.

Margaret: Well, it is called "a discipline"! Hey, my brother is playing at Desperado tonight. Do you want to go?

JP: Sure! I hope he plays that "Bar BQ Fool" song. You can dance the tango or whatever you want to that. Being a nutritionist, I like the irony of the title.

PART V

Cost-Effectiveness and Cost–Benefit Analysis

Chapter 16 gives an overview of cost-effectiveness and cost–benefit analysis. Every year millions of dollars are spent on food and nutrition intervention programs that are designed to improve health. Given that money can always be spent in many different ways, this leads to a natural question: How effective was the program, relative to how much it cost? There are two standard approaches to answering this question: a cost-effectiveness analysis and a cost–benefit analysis. The chapter covers the main questions that must be answered in doing either a cost-effectiveness or cost–benefit analysis. The main formulas in each approach are presented. The pros and cons of each approach are discussed. A hypothetical nutrition intervention program provides context for the discussion.

Chapter 16

Cost-Effectiveness and Cost–Benefit Analysis

Learning Objectives

What you will know by the end of this chapter:

◻ the five main questions you need to answer in doing a cost-effectiveness and cost–benefit analysis;
◻ the definition and components of a cost-identification analysis;
◻ the definition and components of a cost-effectiveness analysis (CEA);
◻ the definition and use of quality-adjusted life-years (QALYs);
◻ the definition and components of a cost–benefit analysis (CBA);
◻ the pros and cons of a CEA versus a CBA; and
◻ why a CEA is preferred over a CBA in nutrition and health interventions.

Opening Conversation

JP: Margaret, Margaret, guess what? My *This City Is Cooking* project got funded! You know, my nutrition education program designed to improve vegetable-cooking skills. I'm so excited! But there's one caveat: they want me to consider doing either a cost-effectiveness or cost–benefit analysis or both. I don't know anything about either one. Do you know anything about them? If so, could you give me an overview?

Margaret: Congratulations! Yeah, I know a little about those methods. Conceptually they are rather straightforward, but the implementation can be difficult. Here's a summary.

What Is the Issue?

Suppose you work for the World Health Organization (WHO). Your boss walks in and says, "You've had some economics. We have two drugs for treating influenza. The first drug costs $20 per shot whereas the second drug costs $22 per shot per patient. We should recommend the first one, right?" Hopefully you would follow-up by saying "Well, assuming they're equally effective, then yes. But if they're not equally effective, then the answer may be no." You continue, "For example, suppose the first drug was only effective at preventing illness in 80% of the cases but the second was effective in 95% of the cases. How much would it cost to prevent the same number of people from getting sick from each drug? Say we wanted to prevent a million people from getting sick. With the first drug we would have to treat 1,250,000 (=1,000,000/0.80) individuals, so the total cost would be $25 million (=1,250,000 × $20). But with the second drug we would only have to treat 1,052,631 (=1,000,000/.95) individuals, for a total cost of about $23 million ($23,167,895 =1,052,631 × $22). So with the second drug you spend about $2 million less and prevent the same number of people from getting sick. In a phrase: Drug 2 is more cost-effective than Drug 1, even though it costs more." The next day your boss gives you a big fat promotion. Congratulations!

The central question being asked in this example is ubiquitous: How effective was the program, relative to how much it cost? The last part of this question is extremely important. As seen, the answer can be completely reversed once it is cast in the context of cost-effectiveness.

The purpose of this chapter is to give a brief introduction to cost-identification analysis, cost-effectiveness analysis (CEA), and cost–benefit analysis (CBA). All three topics are related, and cost-identification analysis is simply calculating the cost of a program. CEA requires a cost-identification analysis, but then takes the total cost and simply converts it to a cost per unit of output or effect. Finally, CBA can be thought of as a type of CEA where the effects of the program have been monetized into a benefits estimate. One of the main themes that will come out of this chapter is that as you move from a cost-identification analysis, to a CEA, to a CBA, you have to make more assumptions.

The Preliminary Questions to Ask and Answer

We hope by this point in the book you realize that one of the most frequently recurring questions in life is this: How should a resource be allocated in order to get the largest benefit? You hear this question posed many different ways: What is the "return on the investment"? What is the "bang for the buck"? To answer this question, you must first answer four preliminary questions:

1. What are the *objectives* in allocating the resource?
2. What are the *options* in allocating the resource?
3. What are the *costs* in allocating the resource?
4. What are the *benefits* in allocating the resource?

Answering the *objectives* question completely requires discipline in thinking and a desire to identify a measurable outcome. To say, "The objective of this program [implying resource allocation] is to improve 'health' " is too vague for evaluation purposes. Is your target some intermediate outcome like changing consumption of some food group? Or is your target some final and ambitious outcome like changing weight? Even if your target is changing nutrition, what does that mean? Are you trying to improve knowledge, attitudes, or consumption? If consumption, what is the target of improved nutrition consumption: Calories? Fat? Saturated fat? Sugar? Fruits? All of these?

Answering the *options* question requires identifying all feasible options for reaching the objectives. Are you going to do some type of educational program? Are you going to change the eating environment? Are you going to provide some direct incentives?

Determining which of the options is feasible requires knowing the cost of each option and thus answering the third question. In some cases answering the *costs* question may be straightforward. For example, suppose your organization has $100,000 to spend on nutrition advertising. Suppose TV advertising cost $200 per minute, Internet advertising $400 per advertisement, and print media $800 per advertisement. You can buy many more TV advertisements than Internet or print media advertisements. Consider now a more complicated example. Suppose you are considering an after-school nutrition education program for children ages 7 through 12. What is the cost for this program? Well, you certainly want to consider the cost to develop the program (e.g., developer's labor time, printed material cost). However, you also want to consider the cost of actually delivering the program, such as a percentage of the teacher's salary (more labor) spent delivering the program. You also want to include other materials used in the actual delivery (e.g., fruits and vegetables used in demonstrations). But what about the gasoline cost associated with the teacher's travel to the delivery site? What about her meal cost if she is in transit during a mealtime? So in some cases the costs can be clear and in other cases a little hazy.

Finally, the *benefits* question is much easier to answer *conceptually* if the objective of the program has been precisely defined. However, *measuring* benefits may be difficult even if conceptually the target or objective is clearly stated. Suppose, for example, the objective of a program or intervention is to increase vegetable consumption in a high school by 10% by the end of the year. What are the "benefits" associated with this? It depends on who you ask. Suppose the program did increase average vegetable consumption by 10%. Is that a benefit to the individual? It is certainly an *effect* of the intervention, but how does the individual benefit from this increase? Supposedly something about the person's health state will improve as a result of the increase in vegetable consumption. How is that to be measured? An increase in the number of years someone is expected to live? A reduction in the amount of medical expenditures for society? All of these are potential benefits. Which is the most appropriate measure?

You can see that doing cost-identification analysis, CEA, and CBA will require you to answer the cost, objectives, and benefits questions rather precisely. Measurement requires clarity in concept translated to a precise quantitative form.

This City Is Cooking: A Hypothetical Nutrition Education Program

For salience, let's construct a hypothetical working example to illustrate the issues involved in cost-identification analysis, CEA, and CBA. Suppose you work at a nonprofit organization hoping to improve the health and nutrition of low-income families in a large city. In reading the literature on barriers to eating vegetables, you have noticed that a lack of vegetable-cooking skills is a major factor. You and your colleagues decide to write a grant entitled *This City Is Cooking*, which will integrate basic nutrition information within the context of a cooking class. The big-picture summary is that you will offer a nine-week cooking course over the summer. The course will meet twice a week on Tuesday and Thursday evening from 6 to 8. The same material will be taught in each of these weekly sessions, allowing families more flexibility. The objective is to provide participating low-income families the skills and therefore confidence to prepare more home-cooked vegetables. You recognize that many people now use some type of tablet device in cooking, so as an incentive to encourage people to participate, you propose to buy all participants an iPad. The iPad will be loaded with nutrition information and a cookbook developed for the class. In addition, each participating family will receive a kitchen starter set that includes pots, pans, cutlery, plates, and measuring cups. The first hour will be a cooking class taught by a professional chef where each family will be at a cooking station and actually cook and eat the meal. The second hour of the class will be nutrition education taught by a registered dietitian. You recognize that one barrier to taking this type of class is that a family may need childcare during the class. Also, some may have to pay for public transportation to get to the class.

You submit the grant with a budget of $40,000. Congratulations! Your grant is approved by the Department of Better Living with one caveat: you must do a cost-identification analysis, CEA, and, if possible, CBA of the program. You agree, though you have never done any one of these before. A colleague recommends you consult this book for an overview, and this is what you find.

Cost-Identification Analysis: Categories and Types

Cost identification is the identification and measurement of the cost associated with some good. Goods in economics are usually broken down into two types: market goods and nonmarket goods. *Market goods* are goods for which there exists a market where the good can be bought and there is an observable price for the good (e.g., an apple, a used car). However, there are numerous goods that are valuable but that are not traded on any formal market, so there is no observable price for the good.[1] Goods of this type are called *nonmarket goods*. Good health or bad

---

[1] Don't confuse "formal" with "legal." A formal market does not have to be a legal market. There are many illegal markets, so-called black markets, that are quite sophisticated and therefore have well-established prices, such as an illegal drug market.

health (e.g., obesity) is a nonmarket good that has an associated cost, but it is not a cost that we can look up on Amazon.com.

Given this market dichotomy, there are then two types of cost-identification analyses. A *market good cost-identification analysis* determines the cost of some market good. A *nonmarket good cost-identification analysis* estimates the cost of some nonmarket good by making numerous assumptions. In this chapter we will focus mainly on nutrition interventions or programs that are designed to improve nutrition in some group of people, which is a nonmarket good. In this type of cost-identification exercise, it is often useful to break down inputs and therefore costs into several different components.

Costs are usually grouped based on four common input classifications and types. The common cost categories are as follows:

1. *Labor costs* (inputs)—The costs associated with human resources used in the production of the good. Obvious examples would be salaries, wages, and benefits.
2. *Capital costs* (inputs)—The costs associated with assets, usually physical, used in the production of the good. Examples would be buildings, cars, and computers.
3. *Material costs* (inputs)—The costs associated with goods specifically required for the production of the good. Examples would be printed material costs, perhaps food models and props used for demonstrations, and foods purchased for cooking lessons.
4. *Utility costs* (inputs)—The costs associated with any type of energy or related inputs used in the production of the good. Examples would be the utility bill for the building or the gasoline cost for travel.

The boundaries between these categories can be fuzzy. For example, one could classify gasoline for travel as a material cost in delivering a program rather than a utility cost. The main thing is that the cost be counted, because in the end all the category costs will be added together to get total cost.

The common cost types are as follows:

i. *Fixed costs* (inputs)—The costs of inputs that will *not* vary with how much of the good is produced. Examples would be a car or a printer.
ii. *Variable costs* (inputs)—The costs of inputs that will vary with how much of the good is produced. Examples would be gasoline used in travel related to delivering a program or paper used for printing materials.
iii. *Direct costs* (*inputs*)—The cost of inputs that are directly related to the production of the good. Examples would be salaries for employees directly related to producing the good or materials used directly in producing the good, such as paper.
iv. *Indirect costs* (*inputs*)—The cost of inputs that are not directly related to the production of the good, but may be considered relevant. These are also sometimes called opportunity costs. Examples would be the value of

a program participant's time while he or she was participating in the program or the value of a lunch that is bought for participants in a program that ran over lunch time.

Fixed and variable costs are mutually exclusive. Direct and indirect costs are mutually exclusive. However, direct costs may be fixed or variable costs and indirect costs may be fixed or variable costs.

Let's return to the hypothetical *This City Is Cooking* project. Table 16.1 shows a breakdown of the various components of the project along with their costs. See the footnote in Table 16.1 for how the numbers are calculated. Importantly, recognize in the context of this example that all variable inputs vary by the number of classes taught and the number of families enrolled. As can be seen, the first six

TABLE 16.1

Cost-Identification Analysis by Type and Category for *This City Is Cooking* Project

Item[a]	Fixed	Variable	Direct	Indirect	Labor	Capital	Materials	Utilities	AMOUNT
Dietitian	×		×		×				$2,250
Chef	×		×		×				$2,250
Participant Recruitment	×		×		×		×		$1,000
Classroom Rental	×		×			×		×	$4,500
Nutrition and Cookbook Development	×		×		×				$3,000
Evaluation Instrument Development	×		×		×				$1,200
Kitchen Starter Kit		×	×				×		$1,500
iPad		×	×				×		$5,000
Food for Classes		×	×				×		$900
Evaluation Instrument Printing		×		×			×		$40
Childcare		×		×	×				$2,700
Public Transport Voucher		×		×				×	$900
									$25,240

[a] Assumptions are as follows. 20 families participate. 15 families have children. 10 need public transport voucher. 9 week program. Dietitian and chef each paid $250 per week for class. Classroom rental is $500/week. Nutrition, cookbook, and evaluation instrument development costs are $3,000, $1,000, and $1,200, respectively. Each family kitchen starter kit and iPad is $75 and $250 respectively. Food purchase per family per week is $5. Evaluation instrument printing is $2 per family. Childcare cost is $20 and public transport voucher is $10 per family per week.

cost items are fixed and will have to be paid regardless of the number of families that enroll.

For these items, essentially contracts have been signed that are independent of the number of families participating. The remaining six items have costs that will vary depending on how many families participate in each line. The total cost of the *This City Is Cooking* project is $25,240.

Cost-Effectiveness Analysis

Let's now turn our attention to CEA. The idea of a CEA is conceptually straightforward. There is some "effect" the program is trying to produce, and the question is this: How much does it cost to produce that effect?

The key formula in a CEA is called the (incremental) *cost-effectiveness ratio* (CER):

$$CER(p_{new}, p_{old}) = \frac{C(p_{new}) - C(p_{old})}{E(p_{new}) - E(p_{old})} \tag{16.1}$$

In Equation 16.1, p stands for the program, so $C(p_i)$ is the cost and $E(p_i)$ the effect associated with program i = old, new. In the frequent case when the old program is the status quo (i.e., no program), then the formula simplifies to

$$CER(p) = \frac{C(p)}{E(p)}. \tag{16.2}$$

Note that Equation 16.2 is simply the average cost per one effect unit produced. If a farmer produces 40,000 peaches at a total cost of $4,000, then the average cost per peach is $0.10 ($4,000/40,000). The same concept applies here. A CER answers the question: How much does it cost per unit of effect produced? The difficulty in many nonmarket settings and program evaluation settings is in determining what is the appropriate effect to measure, and this is why answering the objective question as precisely as possible is so important.

Let's return to the *This City Is Cooking* project. What is the appropriate effect to measure in this case? Remember the goal of the project was to increase vegetable consumption in the participants. Let's suppose you decided to go with a simple pre- and post-program food checklist to measure the change in vegetable consumption. The question you ask is: How frequently do you have vegetables with dinner (other than potatoes) in a week? Possible answers are: less than once per week, two or three times per week, three to five times per week, five to seven times per week. You decide an improvement would be a move from a lower category to a higher category. You then consider the "effect" of the program to be the number of individuals who improved on the vegetable frequency question. At the end of the project you determine that 18 of the 20 families improved their vegetable consumption based on your criterion. You are now ready to calculate your

CER. However, you realize you could also calculate a CER per participant to go along with the CER per improvement.

Table 16.2 gives the relevant CER numbers from the *This City Is Cooking* project. The cost per participant (Column 4) was $1,262. The cost per improvement (Column 5) was $1,402. You find these numbers quite enlightening but at the same time now somewhat unnerving.

Are these numbers high or low? What you really want to do is compare the CER of your program to the CER for some other program. However, without some standardized unit, you cannot determine whether your CER value is high or low. While cost (the numerator) will always be in dollars across programs, the problem is that the effects (denominator) can differ from one program to another. This is especially problematic if different instruments are being used to measure effects or if there is no agreement on the appropriate effects measure.

Quality-Adjusted Life-Years and the Cost Utility Ratio

The standard solution to the effect unit measurement problem is to convert all effects into what are known as quality-adjusted life-years. *Quality-adjusted life-years* (QALYs) is an index for measuring the quantity and quality of remaining years of life for an individual. The quantity part of the formula is based on life expectancy tables and the quality part is based on a scale from 0 to 1. A quality value of 1 means full health and a value of 0 means death. For example, suppose a man has been diagnosed with a disease and is expected to live only two years without any treatment. The first year he will be in full health, but the second year his health will only be at one-third full health. Consequently, his QALYs is $1.0 \times 1 + 0.3 \times 1 = 1.3$ years. Alternatively, suppose he can be completely cured with a treatment and his remaining life expectancy will be 10 years in full health. In this case his QALYs is $1.0 \times 10 = 10$. The difference in the QALYs associated with the treatment is $\Delta QALYs = 8.7 = 10 - 1.3$. The treatment added 8.7 QALYs to this person's life. If all treatment-related costs are $60,000, the CER for the treatment is $60,000 \div 8.7 = \$6,897$. In other words, the treatment cost $6,897 per *additional* QALY.

When QALYs are used in a cost-effectiveness analysis, the resulting analysis is often called a *cost-utility analysis* and the CER a *cost-utility ratio* (CUR). Because the effect is in terms of an objective unit that is common across studies, CURs from different interventions can be compared and ranked. A treatment or intervention with a smaller CUR (i.e., cost per QALY gained) is preferred over a treatment with a higher CUR. Many agencies classify an intervention as cost-effective if its CUR

TABLE 16.2

Total Cost, Effects, and Cost-Effectiveness Ratios for *This City Is Cooking* Project

Total Cost	Number of Participants	Number of Improvements	CER Participants	CER Improvements
$25,240	20	18	$1,262	$1,402

value is less than $50,000, although the method and thresholds are not without debate (e.g., Neumann, Cohen, and Weinstein 2014). Beyond these debates, there is one major limitation of a CEA.

Cost–Benefit Analysis

The major limitation of any CEA, including the CUR, is that it does not tell us the benefits of the intervention. Health interventions are more accurately considered an investment, not just a cost, with expected future benefits. For example, suppose an accountant and a professional baseball player each suffer a torn ligament in their right arm. To simply remove the pain, the most cost-effective treatment may be rest and physical therapy. However, the professional baseball player needs more than just pain relief; he needs completely restored functionality. His arm is his livelihood, so the additional benefits from the surgery outweigh the additional costs. A CBA is a natural extension to a CEA where the benefits of the intervention are also considered.

A CBA takes the effects of an intervention, converts the effects into a dollar value, and then compares the cost(s) to the benefit(s). The costs are the same as the numerator in the CEA. The *benefits* refer to all positive outcomes that can be attributed to the intervention or program measured in dollars. Benefits are usually separated into direct and indirect benefits. *Direct benefits* are the primary positive targeted outcomes associated with the program that accrue to program participants (e.g., lower weight). *Indirect benefits* are any benefits that are not primary targeted benefits associated with the program (e.g., more productivity at work).

Let $C(p)$ and $B(p)$ be the sum of all costs and benefits associated with some intervention or program p, respectively. There are two general formulas used in CBA. The *net benefit* is just the difference between the benefits and the costs:

$$NB(p) = B(p) - C(p): \text{ Net benefits of a program} \qquad (16.3)$$

If the benefits are greater than the costs, the net benefit is positive ($NB > 0$) and worth the cost. A greater net benefit will be preferred to a smaller net benefit. The other standard formula found in CBA is the *benefit–cost ratio*:

$$BCR(p) = B(p) / C(p): \text{ Benefit Cost Ratio of a program} \qquad (16.4)$$

If all benefits are greater than all costs, the benefit–cost ratio will be greater than one ($BCR > 1$). A program is viewed as acceptable when the BCR is greater than one.

The net benefit formula tells the net value of the program, whereas the benefit–cost ratio tells you the relative value of the program—relative to the cost. For example, suppose you are looking at two programs and one has a net benefit value of $10,000 and the other has a net benefit value of $1,000. You are tempted to say that the first program is more valuable, but you do not know the components, the benefits and the costs. Suppose the first one had total benefits of $15,000 and total costs of $5,000 but the second one had total benefits of $1,200 and total costs of $200. The corresponding benefit cost ratios are then $BCR_1 = 3$ and $BCR_2 = 6$.

For every $1 you put in Program 1 you got back $3, but for every $1 you put in Program 2 you got back $6. Program 2 has a higher rate of return or "bang for the buck" than Program 1, so it may be preferred.

The main challenge in doing a CBA in the area of health is measuring the benefits. In the medical intervention literature, the most common way to measure benefits is to use some combination of (1) future medical cost savings, (2) future loss of income avoided due to restored health, and (3) future loss of income avoided due to postponing death.[2]

This City Is Cooking Evaluation: Cost Utility and CBA Issues

Let's return to the *This City Is Cooking* project evaluation. Based on the previous two sections, it seems there may be some advantages to conducting a cost-utility analysis and a CBA. What types of additional questions or information will be needed for these analyses?

Box 16.1 gives a sample of questions that would have to be answered to conduct a cost-utility analysis and a CBA for a food and nutrition intervention. These questions would have to be answered in addition to answering the costs and effects questions encountered earlier. In answering the first five questions, and many others, the goal is to convert the effects of the program into a change in the QALYs for each of the individuals participating. How would you go about answering these daunting questions? Being a scholar, you would consult the literature. Unfortunately, you will find only partial answers to these questions. Consequently, you will have to supplement your literature review with some assumptions in order to achieve the quantitative precision required to implement the measure.

As we discussed in Chapters 1 and 2, improved nutrition will improve health and conceptually therefore will lead to a higher QALY value. However, the difficulty we have also discussed in several places is that the connection among food intake, nutrition, and health is very complex and affected by many factors. If a QALY is going to be used as the effect resulting from a nutrition intervention, then the change in nutrition intake will have to be translated into a numeric change in QALY. Note that in the context of the *This City Is Cooking* project, this would implying converting the reported change in weekly vegetable consumption into a change in the number of QALYs over the individual's entire expected lifespan! Clearly such a conversion can be done, but it would obviously require numerous strong (heroic?) assumptions on behavioral change permanency and the links among food intake, nutrition, and disease for the individual, which are all known to be age- and gender-specific. As the intricacies of the calculations and the assumptions mount, so may skepticism about the actual CUR number obtained.

---

[2] Unfortunately, any one of these three involves numerous assumptions and calculations, including taking into consideration the time value of money and discounting. Given the conclusion we will come to on CBA for nutrition interventions, we do not go into detail on these calculations. In the conclusions we give several references for learning more about CEA and CBA.

BOX 16.1

Sample Questions to Answer for a Cost-Utility and Cost–Benefit Analysis for the *This City Is Cooking* Project

---

Cost Utility Sample Questions (in addition to those already answered)

◘ What diseases are affected by a change in vegetable consumption?

◘ What is the incidence rate of the diseases affected by vegetable consumption?

◘ How many years will the increase in vegetable consumption last?

◘ How many additional years of life are due to the increase in vegetable frequency?

◘ How will the quality of life for each year improve on a scale of 0 to 1?

Cost–Benefit Sample Questions (in addition to the above questions)

◘ What treatment alternatives are avoided by increased vegetable consumption for the diseases identified?

◘ How much does each of the avoided treatment alternatives cost now or sometime within the expected lifespan?

◘ What is the change in the projected present value of lifetime earnings associated with the change in expected lifetime associated with increased vegetable consumption?

What about the CBA? As we hope we've made clear, a CBA is an extension of a CEA and will require converting the effects into some type of dollar benefit. In doing this, the remaining questions in Box 16.1, among others, would have to be answered. Again, one would consult the literature on these questions. Consequently, all the assumptions required to measure the effects for the CEA must now be coupled with assumptions required to convert the effects to a dollar value. So, in doing the CBA, another layer of intricate calculations and assumptions would be added—and perhaps then another layer of skepticism.

The Pros and Cons of CEA and CBA in Nutrition Interventions

At this point your enthusiasm for CEA and CBA may be gone. You may be thinking that in a nutrition intervention program there are simply too many assumptions and the CEA and CBA results are laden with too much uncertainty to be reliable or plausible. However, in this section we want to encourage you not to "throw the baby out with the bath water." There are certainly cons associated with these methods, but there also pros that make them worthy of being added to the list of information about the effectiveness of nutrition interventions. The key is to identify the source of the limitations, be cognizant of these limitations, and work to avoid them or develop ways to reduce them.

Let's start with the major pros and cons of CBA. The major pros are that all values in a CBA are expressed in dollar terms, so there is a standardized unit. A CBA not only measures cost but also tells the benefits associated with those costs and gives a "bang-for-the-buck" estimate via the benefit–cost ratio. The major cons of the CBA are that numerous and often unverifiable assumptions are required about the effects of the intervention, on not only the length of life but the quality of life. Because a dollar value is being placed on a life, which is usually based on existing income or salary levels, rich individuals will be valued more than poor individuals. Therefore a CBA implicitly contains controversial ethical issues. Finally, because a net benefit value is calculated, it identifies an option for optimal resource allocation that may be inconsistent with other goals of the intervention not included in the analysis.

The major pros and cons of CEA are somewhat the reverse of the CBA. The major pros of CEA are that it requires fewer assumptions than a CBA. It avoids the ethical issues associated with placing a dollar value on a life. It places no explicit weight on how resources should be allocated to achieve an effect; rather, it simply provides a measure of the efficient use of resources via the cost per unit of effect. The major cons of CEA are that it does not measure benefits and therefore does not give a "bang-for-the-buck" figure. A CEA does not have single standardized unit.

So given these pros and cons, which approach is recommended? In 1993, the Panel on Cost-Effectiveness in Health and Medicine (PCEHM) was formed by the U.S. Public Health Service to address the growing need for evaluative techniques that could be used in an era of increasing restrictions on health care expenditures. This panel consisted of 13 nongovernmental scientists and scholars who had expertise in CEA and came from several disciplinary backgrounds, ranging from medicine to economics to psychology to sociology. One of the first tasks of the panel was determine whether they would recommend a CBA or CEA approach. As they state:

> [The] health sector has traditionally favored economic analyses that assess cost per unit of health effect, resisting the use of the closely associated technique of cost benefit analysis (CBA), where both costs and benefits are measured in dollars. A number of ethical difficulties ranging from macro issues, such as the effect of valuing the time people spend pursuing medical treatment according to their wages [an indirect cost], are already embedded in CEA. CBA adds an additional difficulty in that it presumes to put a dollar figure on the value of human life and uses controversial methods to do so. The panel has shared the dominant bias of the health sector—that monetizing the price of life in these ways introduces ethical concerns that are avoided by CEA, albeit at the sacrifice of generalizability. (Gold et al. 1996, p. xxii)

Given this assessment of CEA relative to CBA, the main limitation of applying a CEA to a nutrition intervention is not the concept; the problem is the lack of an appropriate standardized effect measure. In the context of medical treatment interventions, the targeted outcome is an extension of life and improvement in the quality of life, and this is what the QALY measures. In the cost-effectiveness literature, a nutrition intervention is an intermediate or preventive intervention that is targeting an intermediate outcome: improved nutrition. Intermediate targets need their own standardized effects measurements that are designed to measure the targeted outcome. As the distance between the targeted intervention outcome (e.g., improved nutrition) and the measurement outcome (e.g., QALY) increases, the number of required assumptions cascades and the level of confidence in the analysis quickly erodes. All of this suggests that the development of a standardized nutrition intervention effects measure would overcome the main limitation of a CEA in nutrition intervention applications. If some index, for example the Healthy Eating Index, could be agreed upon for measuring change in nutrition quality, then this information could be collected as part of any nutrition intervention. Thus, all nutrition interventions would have a standard basis for comparison via a CEA.

Conclusions and Some Empirical Applications

This chapter provided an overview of CEA and CBA. Both are designed to provide useful information in addressing a resource allocation problem. The CEA yields a cost per unit of output produced called the CER. The CER is therefore an efficiency measure of the resources spent but does not say anything about benefits received. As long as CERs use a standardized effect across studies, then they can be compared. Alternatively, the CBA extends the CEA to include benefits, where the benefits are measured in a monetary unit as well (e.g., dollars). The CBA provides two common measures: the net benefit, which is just the difference in the benefits and the cost, and the benefit–cost ratio. The benefit–cost ratio is a measure of the "bang for the buck" of the intervention, and a benefit–cost ratio greater than one is considered good. Both the CEA and CBA are conceptually sound and useful frameworks for thinking through resource allocation problems. However, empirically, each has pros and cons. The CEA appears to have more pros than cons and is the measure of choice in most health applications. The main limitation of applying the CEA in nutrition interventions is the lack of a standardized measure of effects, and this is a fruitful area for future research.

The literature on CEA and CBA is quite voluminous in the medical treatment area but sparser in the nutrition intervention area. The program that has received the most attention in terms of CEA and CBA is the Adult Expanded Food and Nutrition Program (A-EFNEP). Most of these studies have been state-level CBAs and followed the methodology of the original Virginia study in 1996 (Rajgopal et al. 2002). Across studies and therefore states, the benefit–cost ratios of the A-EFNEP have ranged from $3.62 (Oregon: Schuster et al. 2003) to $8.34 (California: Joy, Pradhan, and Goldman 2006), $9.58 (New York: Dollahite, Kenkel, and Thompson 2008), and $10.64 (Virginia: Rajgopal et al. 2002). All of these numbers indicate a very good "bang for the buck." Given the documented numerous assumptions going into a CBA, and the fact that these are different states at different time periods, these numbers are surprisingly consistent, though that may be due to the fact that they all followed the same methodological approach. Two studies have conducted a CEA and calculated the CER per QALY. Dollahite, Kenkel, and Thompson (2008) calculated the CER per QALY for the A-EFNEP in New York to be $20,863. Following Dollahite et al. (2008) very closely, Baral et al. (2013) used national-level data on the EFNEP and calculated the CER per QALY (i.e., CUR) for each state during the 2000–2006 period. They found a great deal of variability in the CURs across states, ranging from a low of $7,389 (Texas) to a high of $101,695 (Mississippi). The median CUR value was $22,904. All but three states (Mississippi, South Carolina, and West Virginia) had CUR values below the $50,000 cutoff, indicating the EFNEP is cost-effective. As Baral et al. (2013) discussed, even if some of the assumptions required to do the analysis are questionable, given the fact that all states are evaluated using the same technique and effect measure, the results are still useful for identifying which states are relatively more cost-efficient.

In closing, the chapter is meant as only an introduction. There are many issues we did not discuss, such as time discounting and sensitivity analysis, and the interested reader should consult one of the many good books on conducting CEA and CBA in health for in-depth coverage (e.g., Gold et al. 1996; Muennig 2007).

The Proposal

JP: I see what you mean. Conceptually both the cost-effectiveness and cost–benefit analyses are very intuitive and straightforward. However, as you say, the devil is in the implementation details. Based on this discussion, and pardon the word play, but it seems like the benefits don't outweigh the costs of doing a cost–benefit analysis. I think I can do a cost-effectiveness analysis, but I'll have to decide what the appropriate effect measurement will be. I'm leaning toward some type of pre-test and post-test design with something like the Healthy Eating Index, but I'll have to research it some more. Thanks, Margaret. We've known each other for about a year now, and I don't know what I would do without you. In fact, I want to talk to you about that.

Margaret: What?

JP: What I would do without you. I don't want to do anything without you. It's as plain as economics: the benefits with you would far exceed the costs.

Margaret: And as important as nutrition. I feel exactly the same way.

APPENDIX

Economic Methodology 101

*Science is built upon facts as a house is built upon stones, but an
accumulation of facts is no more science than an accumulation of stones
is a house.*

—POINCARÉ (1905, P. 158)

As indicated in the book preface, economics is a systematic framework for analyzing economic phenomena. But what differentiates the economic approach generally from some other disciplines?

Economists are trying to do the same thing all scientists are trying to do: understand and explain phenomena. All sciences use some form of the scientific method—systematic observation, measurement, organization, synthesis, hypothesis formulation, experimentation, data analysis, hypothesis testing, and modification. However, the particulars of the scientific process vary a great deal within and across disciplines. Even within a discipline, there may be different terms for the same concept or the same term for different concepts. More problematic, across disciplines the terminology and methods may differ so much that a person in one discipline may not even recognize another discipline as a science. Thus, much of the miscommunication that occurs within and especially across disciplines stems from scientific language and grammar differences (Kuhn 1993).

One of the main goals of this book is to help bridge the communication gap between economists and health scientists. Good communication begins with precision in terminology and making sure everyone is starting from familiar ground. Consequently, in this appendix we first review the main conceptual components of all sciences and then identify the main characteristic of economic analysis that we believe helps explain the structure of the economic approach. Economists have been discussing the appropriate methodology (logic of methods) for their subject for a long time, and most of the fundamental insights were made very early on by John Stuart Mill (1950). This appendix is a watered-down summary of Davis (2000, 2004), and the interested reader should consult those articles for more details and many more references.

Science Conceptual Components and Economic Methodology

Science is disciplined curiosity: why does this phenomena (e.g., cancer, obesity) occur? In answering this question, the scientist identifies the *effect* variable(s) of interest (e.g., abnormal cell growth or higher obesity incidence) and then postulates some *cause* variable(s) of the effect. So at the most basic level the scientist partitions all the variables in the world into two sets:

(i)   the relevant set (effects of interest and their causes) and
(ii) the irrelevant set (all other variables).

This variable partitioning is the first step in creating a theory of the relationship between cause and effect variables. A *theory* is therefore an abstraction of reality that explains some phenomenon with a subset of selected causal variables. Most theories, especially in economics, will identify multiple causes. The theory is an abstraction because by definition it omits some possible variables as explanations. For example, in the absence of friction, Galileo's theory of falling objects says that all objects fall to the earth at a constant rate of acceleration of 32 feet per second. The effect of interest is the rate of acceleration of a falling object, the single cause is gravity, and all other variables, with the exception of friction, are not important, such as the color or smell of the object. The theory has therefore invoked an assumption about what is important and what is not important.

An *assumption* is a statement that is presumed true without proof (e.g., the object's color does not matter). There are always two types of assumptions used in theories: implicit and explicit.

Implicit assumptions are effectively this: if the theory did not mention something (e.g., a variable), then it is assumed to be irrelevant or not changing. Alternatively, if a variable is included in the theory but is not the focus (e.g., friction), then an explicit assumption is usually made that this variable is assumed to be constant or not changing in order to isolate the effect of the variable of interest (e.g., gravity). Rather than try to list all other variables assumed to be irrelevant or held constant, an impossible task, it is standard in economics to use the encompassing qualifier assumption *ceteris paribus*. *Ceteris paribus* is a Latin term literally meaning all else constant, but it is probably better translated as ignoring (perhaps for the moment) the effects of other possible causes. *All* sciences use the *ceteris paribus* assumption, even if it is not stated. In fact, unfortunately it is often forgotten in economics, but this is somewhat understandable as it can get quite redundant to qualify every statement with *ceteris paribus*.

Based on the assumptions about the underlying causal and effect mechanism and the *ceteris paribus* assumption, the laws of the theory are derived. A *theoretical law* is a derived statement of a specific type of relationship between causal and effect variables. A *hypothesis* is just an observational representation of a theoretical law. If a hypothesis has been tested and confirmed in a variety of settings, then it may be called an *empirical law*. The terms *theory*, *hypothesis*, and *law* are often used interchangeably in scientific discussions.

The Languages of Science and Insights from Math

A theory is nothing but a story about the relationship between variables. Obviously, stories can be told in different languages. Scientists use three languages to tell stories: (i) a text or spoken language (e.g., English, French), (ii) a graphical language (e.g., plots, charts), and (iii) a mathematical language (e.g., algebra, calculus, statistics). Each language has advantages and disadvantages. None is a panacea. Text is easy to use and good for nuanced and imprecise claims, but it is not good for measurement, precision, and manipulation to uncover further logical implications. Graphs are very good for quickly conveying a lot of two-dimensional relationships but are not very good for higher-dimensional relationships. Math is extremely good at representing very precisely possibly intricate multidimensional relationships and manipulating these relationships to uncover unanticipated implications, but math is the hardest of these languages to master and comprehend. Fortunately, the concepts presented in this book require fluency in math only at the middle-school level. And middle-school math is the most efficient, most precise, and clearest way to present the main concepts of this book.

Suppose we have some phenomenon (effect) Y that is determined by two causal variables, $X1$ and $X2$, by the equation

$$Y = 200 + 100X_1 - 10X_2 \tag{A.1}$$

Don't worry what the variables are at this point. Just focus on understanding the concepts. To keep it simple, suppose X_1 and X_2 can take on two possible values: 0 and 1. All the possible values of Y associated with X_1 and X_2 are then

X1	X2	Y
0	0	200
0	1	190
1	0	300
1	1	290

There are three important points to be recognized by this simple example:

1. *Effects of causes are not causes of effects.* Huh? One of the first things we notice is that the contribution of each causal variable to Y is very different. As X_1 increases by 1, Y will increase by 100 (e.g., rows 1 and 3), but as X_2 increases by 1, Y decreases by only 10 (e.g., rows 1 and 2). Thus the "effects of the causes" are different. So while the causes of the effect (Y) are X_1 and X_2, the effects of the causes (100 and −10) are different. Succinctly stated, *effects of causes are not causes of effects* (Holland 1986).

2. *Some causes are more important than others.* This is just a corollary to #1. In science we usually seek to isolate a single effect (e.g., gravity). However, if there are multiple causes (e.g., gravity and friction), then some causes usually will be more important (have a larger impact on Y) than others, and our desire is to isolate the most important causes. In the above case, X_1 is more important than X_2 in terms of Y.

3. *The effect of one variable may accentuate or attenuate the effect of another variable.* Note from the above table that the effect of X_1 would be greater if X_2 did not change (e.g., compare the change from row 1 to 3 with the change from row 1 to 4).

4. *An effect can be relevant without being universal, and an effect can be universal without being relevant (the universal vs. relevance principle).* This is an implication of the first three. It is not immediately obvious from the table but becomes apparent with a little explanation. In most cases we tend to think of causal variables as always active and never dormant. However, often it is the case that an important causal variable can remain unchanged for a long time and then when it changes it overwhelms some other effect(s). Indeed, isn't this what happens when someone contracts a terminal disease? For example, suppose X_2 is switched on and off daily in this process but X_1 is activated only monthly. In terms of the change in Y, X_1 is very relevant but not universal, whereas X_2 is universal but not very relevant (relative to X_1). There are numerous examples of the need to make these distinctions (e.g., a natural disaster, wartime vs. peacetime, etc.).

Models and the Importance of *Ceteris Paribus* in Economic Analysis

Of course, if we actually knew the Equation A.1, we would not need to look at any data as we already know the relationship between the variables. Suppose all we observe are the values of Y, X_1, and X_2. Furthermore, suppose our real interest is in isolating the effect of X_1 on Y. How can we do this? Usually the scientist will begin by specifying a *model*, which is often a graphical or mathematical representation of the theory.[1] Models are extremely prevalent in economics, but we first need to be very clear on distinguishing the conceptual from the empirical. Most scientists will agree on the conceptual side of the ledger; most of the differences come on the empirical side.

What we want to know, but do not know, are the values of the effects of X_1 and X_2. Thus the scientist may start with a model like

$$Y = \beta_1 X_1 + \beta_2 X_2 : \text{Linear model} \tag{A.2}$$

---

[1] As Poirier (1995, p. 585) has stated, "a true model is an oxymoron if there ever was one." One can think of a true model as one that fits the data perfectly, and in some disciplines, such as physics, the degree of error in models is so small that they may be considered effectively true. This is not the case in social sciences, and hence Poirier's comment.

However, because the scientist wants to know how Y changes as X_1 changes by 1 unit, it is therefore more convenient to write this in its change form as

$$\Delta Y = \beta_1 \Delta X_1 + \beta_2 \Delta X_2 : \text{Linear model in change form} \qquad (A.3)$$

where Δ indicates change. In words, the change in Y is determined by β_1 times the change in X_1 plus β_2 times the change in X_2. With the focus on X_1, the scientist wants to determine the value of β_1 but how?

Let's consider two scenarios: (i) a controlled experimental setting and (ii) a noncontrolled experimental (observational) setting. In the controlled experimental setting the scientist recognizes that X_2 may be important and so designs an experiment where X_2 can have no effect on the outcome of Y, or equivalently stated mathematically $\Delta X_2 = 0$. The scientist then changes X_1 by 1 unit and observes a change in Y of 100, or more succinctly, the data are $\Delta X_2 = 0$, $\Delta X_1 = 1$, and $\Delta Y = 100$, and so from Equation A.3, $\Delta Y = 100 = \beta_1$ and the desired effect is isolated. Note as a consequence of the design of the experiment, the scientist does not have to worry about the effect of X_2 and so is effectively working with the partial model

$$\Delta Y = \beta_1 \Delta X_1 : \text{Experimental model} \qquad (A.4)$$

Now consider the observational setting where the scientist cannot conduct a controlled experiment but just observes the data $\Delta X_1 = 1$, $\Delta X_2 = 1$, and $\Delta Y = 90$ (rows 1 and 4). Substituting these values into Equation A.3 yields $\Delta Y = 90 = \beta_1 + \beta_2$. Is the scientist to conclude the effect of a change in X_1 on Y is 90 (i.e., $\beta_1 = 90$)? Of course not; part of the effect on Y may be due to X_2 (i.e., β_2). So in the observational setting the scientist needs to use the more general model in Equation A.3— $\Delta Y = \beta_1 \Delta X_1 + \beta_2 \Delta X_2$—and then couple this with an assumption or information about $\beta_2 \Delta X_2$. The observational setting therefore requires a more general model, and sophisticated mathematical and statistical techniques are used to substitute for experimental control to isolate the effect of X_1. But both approaches are trying to achieve the same objective: isolate the effect of X_1. In more general terms, as we indicated above, there will be variables, such as X_2, that can offset the effect of the variable of interest, and these can be categorized many ways and by many names, but a common general name is *concomitants*. Because of concomitants, the word *tendency* is often used to describe the effects of a variable of interest that exist but may be offset by another variable (Cartwright 1989; Mill 1950).

One of the most distinguishing features of economics, in comparison to other disciplines (e.g., chemistry, biology), is that the subject matter does not easily lend itself to controlled experiments for multiple reasons. Yes, economists do experiments and increasingly so, but much economic analysis is still based on observational data, which means concomitants are always a concern when trying to draw correct inferences. Consequently, to avoid faulty inferences, the economist must recognize, use, and develop a more comprehensive framework for analysis and then judiciously use the *ceteris paribus* assumption to conceptually isolate effects.

This framework and discussion is also useful for understanding the important difference between internal validity and external validity. *Internal validity* refers to a property of an analysis where the results are due only to a change in the variable(s) of interest and not some other factor. *External validity* refers to a property of an analysis where the results of an analysis can be generalized to other settings where there may not be control over other factors. Thus, within a vacuum, Galileo's theory of falling objects is internally valid, but it is not externally valid when friction is not accounted for in the explanation (i.e., all objects do not fall at the same rate in an external environment due to friction). These distinctions are useful for comparing experimental and observational approaches because each has advantages and disadvantages. Well-designed experimental studies will isolate the effect of interest and will be internally valid, but because they are holding concomitants constant they *may* not be externally valid. Alternatively, because observational studies cannot control concomitants, it can be difficult to isolate the effect of a cause, but the finding *may* be externally valid because concomitants are allowed to have an influence as well.

Moderators and Mediators

As indicated, most phenomena have multiple causes, so another way of classifying variables is useful for describing the relationship between variables. Often it will be the case that some variable will moderate (either accentuate or attenuate) the effect of another variable; such a variable is called a *moderator*. For example, if we are trying to explain weight in terms of height, we know that females generally weigh less than males for the same height, so gender moderates the effect of height on weight. Alternatively, a *mediator* is a variable that causal or moderating variables operate through. For example, one may claim that many factors can lead to comfort eating, such as loss of a job, loss of a girlfriend, or some other emotional event. However, it would probably be recognized that these are all causes of depression, and depression may be the real cause, so these variables just mediate through the depression variable.

Mathematically the mediating and moderating variables could underlie Equation A.1 as follows. Suppose the variable Y is really determined by a mediating variable M and X_2, so the underlying relationship is

$$Y = 200 + 50M - 10X_2 \tag{A.5}$$

However, the mediating variable is actually determined by X_1, and that relationship is moderated by a variable D such that

$$M = 2X_1 + 2X_1 D \tag{A.6}$$

Substituting Equation A.6 into A.5 yields

$$Y = 200 + 100X_1 + 100X_1D - 10X_2 \qquad\qquad (A.7)$$

So how Y responds to X_1 now depends on the level of D. The table below shows how this would change some of the results from the previous table.

X1	X2	D	Y
0	0	0	200
1	0	1	400

So when $D = 1$, the effect of X_1 is accentuated from 100 to 200. Mediating and moderating variables can interact in numerous ways; consult Baron and Kenny (1986) for more details.

Positive versus Normative Analysis

In much of science, especially social sciences, two distinct questions and therefore answers are often conflated:

1. *What is* the effect of an intervention, policy, or program?
2. *What should be* the intervention, policy, or program implemented?

The first question can be answered without answering the second question and vice versa. Economists use the terms "positive" and "normative" analysis to distinguish between analyses that answer these two questions. A *positive analysis* is an analysis that just states what is or more specifically analyzes (e.g., predicts) the effects of a policy variable—where the term "policy" is being used to include interventions or programs as well. A *normative analysis* is an analysis that states what should be. A normative analysis will usually conduct a positive analysis but then also give an argument for why the policy should be pursued. Although of course any type of analysis involves assumptions, a positive analysis is usually characterized as being agnostic on whether the policy should be implemented and just is stating the expected facts and is characterized as objective. Alternatively, a normative analysis is not agnostic and will usually take some position on the policy being implemented, either criticizing or defending it, and thus it goes beyond stating the expected facts and is considered subjective.

For example, suppose two economists are asked to evaluate the impact of a 20% sugar-sweetened beverage tax on caloric intake. Positive Economist analyzes the tax and determines the tax will decrease caloric intake by 5% per person over a year and says nothing else. Normative Economist comes to the same conclusion but then goes on to say the tax *should* be implemented because it will improve people's health and that is the most important thing to consider. However, an alternative normative economist may analyze the problem and come to the same conclusion but then also consider the impact on the sugar beverage industry and claim the tax should not be implemented because it will decrease profits and therefore jobs in the beverage industry. The main point of making this distinction is that a positive economic analysis of a policy can be done without endorsing or rejecting a policy. The endorsement or rejection is a separate question, and politicians are usually responsible for answering those questions. Of course, economists are often asked to provide their subjective opinion on whether or not a policy *should* be implemented, but that is a different question from the expected fact question: What will the anticipated effect of the policy be?

Conclusions

Science tends to focus on the effects of one variable at a time, but unfortunately most phenomena have multiple causes. Scientists therefore must use conceptual and empirical techniques to isolate the effect of interest, and economics is not different. Most of this book communicates *positive* economic analysis with a graphical and mathematical language that will evaluate how an effect variable will change as some other cause variables change *ceteris paribus*. The analysis is then extended to explore the impact of relaxing the *ceteris paribus* assumption in various directions. The predominant domain of economic analysis is that of a noncontrolled environment, and we hope this brief appendix helps explain why this sort of setting requires a structured and sequential approach to help minimize drawing faulty inferences. Candidly, conceptually the approach is rather straightforward, but empirically it is immensely challenging. Much of science is the business of quantifying concepts. The quantification techniques used in economics are far beyond the scope of this book, but the concepts are not. We must know what we are trying to measure (the concepts) before we can measure it.

REFERENCES

Alonso, R., I. Brocas, and J. Carrillo (2014). "Resource Allocation in the Brain." *Rev Econ Stud* **81**(2): 501–534.

Alston, J., D. Sumner, and S. Vosti (2008). "Farm Subsidies and Obesity in the United States: National Evidence and International Comparisons." *Food Policy* **33**(6): 470–479.

American Cancer Society (2014*). Cancer Facts & Figures*. Atlanta, GA: American Cancer Society.

American Diabetes Association (2014). "Statistics About Diabetes." Retrieved November 11, 2014, from http://www.diabetes.org/diabetes-basics/statistics/?loc=db-slabnav.

Andreoni, J., and C. Sprenger (2012). "Risk Preferences Are Not Time Preferences." *Am Econ Rev* **102**(7): 3357–3376.

Andreyeva, T., M. Long, and K. Brownell (2010). "The Impact of Food Prices on Consumption: A Systematic Review of Research on the Price Elasticity of Demand for Food." *Am J Public Health* **100**(2):216–222.

Andreyeva, T., I. Kelly, and J. Harris (2011). "Exposure to Food Advertising on Television: Associations with Children's Fast Food and Soft Drink Consumption and Obesity." *Econ Hum Biol* **9**: 221–233.

Antonides, G., and L. Cramer (2013). "Impact of Limited Cognitive Capacity and Feelings of Guilt and Excuse on the Endowment Effects for Hedonic and Utilitarian Types of Foods." *Appetite* **68**: 51–55.

Appelhans, B., M. Waring, K. Schneider, S. Pagoto, M. DeBiasse, M. Whited, and E. Lynch (2012). "Delay Discounting and Intake of Ready-to-Eat and Away-From-Home Foods in Overweight and Obese Women." *Appetite* **59**: 576–584.

Appelhans, B., K. Woolf, S. Pagoto, K. Schneider, M. Whited, and R. Liebman (2011). "Inhibiting Food Reward: Delay Discounting, Food Reward Sensitivity, and Palatable Food Intake in Overweight and Obese Women." *Obesity* **19**: 2175–2182.

Bachus, J., and J. Otten (2015). *Healthy Nutrition: From Farm to Fork.* Washington, DC: President's Council on Fitness, Sports, and Nutrition, p. 16.

Baral, R., G. Davis, S. Blake, W. You, and E. Serrano (2013). "Using National Data to Estimate Average Cost Effectiveness of EFNEP Outcomes by State/Territory." *J Nutr Educ Behav* **45**(2): 183–187.

Baron, R., and D. Kenny (1986). "The Moderator–Mediator Variable Distinction in Social Psychological Research: Conceptual, Strategic, and Statistical Considerations." *J Person Soc Psych* **51**(6): 1173.

Basmann, R. (1956). "A Theory of Demand with Variable Consumer Preferences." *Econometrica* **24**(1): 47–58.

Bassett, M., T. Dumanovsky, C. Huang, L. Silver, C. Young, and C. Nonas (2007). "Purchasing Behavior and Calorie Information at Fast-Food Chains—New York City." *Am J Public Health* **98**: 1457–1459.

Batra, R., and O. Ahtola (1991). "Measuring the Hedonic and Utilitarian Sources of Consumer Attitudes." *Mkting Letters* **2**(April): 159–170.

Becker, G. (1962). "Irrational Behavior and Economic Theory." *J Pol Econ* **70**(1): 1–13.

Becker, G. (1965). "A Theory of the Allocation of Time." *Econ J* 75(299):493–517.

Becker, G. (1985). "Human Capital, Effort, and the Sexual Division of Labor." *J Labor Econ* **3**(1): S33–S58.

Becker, G. (1993). "Nobel Lecture: The Economic Way of Looking at Behavior." *J Pol Econ* **101**(3): 385–409.

Becker, G. (2008). *Economic Theory*. New York: Aldine Transaction.

Beghin, J., and H. Jensen (2008). "Farm Policies and Added Sugars in US Diets." *Food Policy* **33**(6): 480–488.

Bentham, J. (1963). *An Introduction to the Principles of Morals and Legislation*. New York: Hafner.

Berner, Y., F. Stern, Z. Polyak, and Y. Dror (2001). "Dietary Intake Analysis in Institutionalized Elderly: A Focus on Nutrient Density." *J Nutr Health and Aging* **6**(4): 237–242.

Berridge, K.C., Ho, C.Y., Richard, J.M., and DiFeliceantonio, A.G. (2010). "The Tempted Brain Eats: Pleasure and Desire Circuits in Obesity and Eating Disorders." *Brain Res* **1950**: 43–64.

Bertalanffy, L. (1979). *General System Theory*. New York: George Braziller.

Beshara, M., A. Hutchinson, and C. Wilson (2010). "Preparing Meals Under Time Stress. The Experience of Working Mothers." *Appetite* **55**: 625–700.

Bezerra, I., C. Curioni, and R. Sichieri (2012). "Association Between Eating Out of Home and Body Weight." *Nutr Rev* **70**(2): 65–79.

Bickel, W., R. Yi, R. Landes, P. Hill, and C. Baxter (2010). "Remember the Future: Working Memory Training Decreases Delay Discounting Among Stimulant Addicts." *Biol Psychiat* **69**: 260–265.

Birch, L., J. Savage, and J. Fisher (2015). "Right Sizing Prevention. Food Portion Size Effects on Children's Eating and Weight." *Appetite* **88**: 11–16.

Blisard, N., H. Stewart, and D. Jolliffe (2004). *Low-Income Households' Expenditures On Fruits and Vegetables*. U.S. Department of Agriculture, Economic Research Service, pp. 1–2.

Block, J., and W. Willett (2013). "Taxing Sugar-Sweetened Beverages: Not A 'Holy Grail' But A Cup At Least Half Full." *Int J Health Policy Mgmnt* **1**(2): 183–185.

Bragulat, V., M. Dzemidzic, C. Bruno, C. Cox, T. Talvage, R. Considine, and D. Kareken (2010). "Food-Related Odor Probes of Brain Reward Circuits During Hunger: A Pilot fMRI Study." *Obesity* **18**: 1566–1571.

Brocas, I., and J. Carrillo (2008). "The Brain As A Hierarchical Organization." *Amer Econ Rev* **98**(4):1312-1346.

Brownell, K., and T. Frieden (2009). "Ounces of Prevention—The Public Policy Case for Taxes on Sugared Beverages." *N Engl J Med* **360**(18): 1805–1808.

Bruno, N., M. Martani, C. Corsini, and C. Oleari (2013). "The Effect of the Color Red on Consuming Food Does Not Depend on Achromatic (Michelson) Contrast and Extends to Rubbing Cream on the Skin." *Appetite* **71**: 307–313.

Bruyneel, S., S. Dewitte, K. Vohs, and L. Warlop (2006). "Repeated Choosing Increases Susceptibility to Affective Product Features." *J Res Mkting* **23**: 215–225.

Bureau of Labor Statistics, Consumer Expenditure Survey (2012). "Quintiles of Income Before Taxes. Table 1101." Retrieved Summer 2014 from http://www.bls.gov/cex/2012/combined/quintile.pdf.

Bureau of Labor Statistics, Inflation and Prices (2014). "All Consumers Price Index Foods and Beverages." Retrieved Summer 2014 from http://www.bls.gov/data/.

Bureau of Labor Statistics, American Time Use Survey (2014). "Civilian Noninstitutional Population Age 15 and Over, Table A-1." Retrieved Summer 2014 from http://www.bls.gov/tus/#tables.

Bureau of Labor Statistics, Employment (2014). "Labor Force Statistics,, Labor Force Participation Rates by Gender." Retrieved Summer 2014 from http://www.bls.gov/data/.

Caldwell, C., and S. Hibbert (2002). "The Influence of Music Tempo and Musical Preference on Restaurant Patrons' Behavior." *Psychol Market* **19**(11): 895–917.

Camerer, C., G. Loewenstein, and D. Prelec (2005). "Neuroeconomics: How Neuroscience Can Inform Economics." *J Econ Lit* **43**: 9–64.

Campos, S., J. Doxey, and D. Hammond (2011). "Nutrition Labels On Pre-Packaged Foods: A Systematic Review." *Public Health Nutr* **14**(8): 1496–1506.

Canning, P. (2011). *A Revised and Expanded Food Dollar Series, A Better Understanding of Our Food Costs.* U.S. Department of Agriculture, p. 114.

Caplan, B. (2003). "Stigler–Becker Versus Myers–Briggs: Why Preference-Based Explanations Are Scientifically Meaningful and Empirically Important." *J Econ Behav Org* **50**(4): 391–405.

Carbone, E., and J. Zoellner (2012). "Nutrition and Health Literacy: A Systematic Review to Inform Nutrition Research and Practice." *J Acad Nutr Diet* **112**(2): 254–265.

Carlson, A., and E. Frazao (2012). *Are Healthy Foods Really More Expensive?* U.S. Department of Agriculture, Washington, DC, p. 96.

Cartwright, N. (1980). "The Truth Doesn't Explain Much." *Am Philos Quart* **17**(2): 159–163.

Cartwright, N. (1989). *Nature's Capacities and Their Measurements.* Oxford: Oxford University Press.

Centers for Disease Control and Prevention (2012). "Increasing Prevalence of Diagnosed Diabetes—United States and Puerto Rico, 1995–2010." *Morbidity and Mortality Weekly Report (MMWR)* **61**(45): 918–921.

Centers for Disease Control and Prevention (2013). "Vital Signs: Avoidable Deaths From Heart Disease, Stroke, and Hypertensive Disease—United States, 2001–2010." *Morbidity and Mortality Weekly Report (MMWR)* **62**(35): 721–727.

Centers for Disease Control and Prevention, Division of Nutrition, Physical Activity, and Obesity. (2015). "About Child and Teen BMI." Retrieved July 1, 2015, from http://www.cdc.gov/healthyweight/assessing/bmi/childrens_bmi/about_childrens_bmi.html.

Centers for Disease Control and Prevention, National Center for Health Statistics (2014). Data Brief 178: Mortality in the United States, 2013. *Data table for Figure 3. Number of deaths, percentage of total deaths, and age-adjusted death rates for the 10 leading causes of death in 2013: United States, 2012–2013.* N. V. S. System.

Chabris, C., D. Laibson, C. Morris, J. Schuldt, and D. Taubinsky (2008). "Individual Laboratory-Measured Discount Rates Predict Field Behavior." *J Risk Uncertain* **37**: 237–269.

Chabris, C., D. Laibson, C. Morris, J. Schuldt, and D. Taubinsky (2009). "The Allocation of Time in Decision-Making." *J Eur Econ Assoc* **7**(2–3): 628–637.

Chandler, A. (2015). Is Fast Food Healthier Than Chipotle? *The Atlantic.* http://www.theatlantic.com/health/archive/2015/02/is-fast-food-better-than-chipotle/385589/

Chou, S., I. Rashad, and M. Grossman (2008). "Food Restaurant Advertising on Television and its Influence on Childhood Obesity." *J Law Econ* **51**(4): 599–618.

Christian, T., and I. Rashad (2009). "Trends in U.S. Food Prices." *Econ Hum Biol* 7: 113–120.

Cohen, D., and S. Babey (2012). "Contextual Influences on Eating Behaviours: Heuristic Processing and Dietary Choices." *Obesity Rev* **13**: 766–779.

Coleman-Jensen, A., C. Gregory, and A. Singh (2014). *Household Food Security in the United States in 2013. A report summary from the Economic Research Service, U.S. Department of Agriculture.*

Conklin, D. (1991). *Objectives, Decision Modes, and the Process of Choice.* New York: Cambridge University Press

Courtemanche, C., G. Heutel, and P. McAlvanah (2015). "Impatience, Incentives and Obesity." *Econ J* **125**(582): 1–31.

Cramer, L., and G. Antonides (2011). "Endowment Effects For Hedonic and Utilitarian Food Products." *Food Qual Prefer* **22**(1): 3–10.

Crifo, P., and V. Forget (2015). "The Economics of Corporate Social Responsibility: A Firm-Level Perspective Survey." *J Econ Surveys* **29**(1): 112–130.

Crook, C. (2005). "The Good Company. The Movement For Corporate Social Responsibility Has Won the Battle of Ideas." *The Economist* **374**(8410): 3–4.

Crouch, M. (2014). "50 Supermarket Tricks You Still Fall For." *Reader's Digest.* 185(February): 177–179.

Curley, S., S. Eraker, and J. Yates (1984). "An Investigation of Patient's Reactions to Therapeutic Uncertainty." *Med Decis Making* 4: 501.

Darmon, N., M. Darmon, M. Maillot, and A. Drewnowski (2005). "A Nutrient Density Standard for Vegetables and Fruits: Nutrients Per Calorie and Nutrients Per Unit Cost." *J Am Diet Assoc* **105**(12): 1881–1887.

Darmon, N., and A. Drewnowski (2008). "Does Social Class Predict Diet Quality?" *Am J Clin Nutr* **87**(5): 1107–1117.

Davis, G. (2000). "A Semantic Interpretation of Haavelmo's Structure of Econometrics." *Econ and Phil* **16**(02): 205–228.

Davis, G. (2004). "The Structure of Models: Understanding Theory Reduction and Testing with a Production Example." *J Agr and Res Econ* **29**(1): 65–78.

Davis, G. (2014). "Food At Home Production and Consumption: Implications For Nutrition Quality and Policy." *Rev Econ Household* **12**(3): 565–588.

Davis, G., and A. Carlson (2015). "The Inverse Relationship Between Food Price and Energy Density: Is It Spurious?" *Public Health Nutr* **18**(6): 1091–1097.

Davis, G., and W. You (2010a). "The Time Cost of Food at Home: General and Food Stamp Participant Profiles." *Appl Econ* **42**(20): 2537–2552.

Davis, G., and W. You (2010b). "The Thrifty Food Plan Is Not Thrifty When Labor Cost Is Considered." *J Nutr* **140**(4): 854–857.

Davis, G., and W. You (2011). "Not Enough Money or Not Enough Time to Satisfy the Thrifty Food Plan? A Cost Difference Approach for Estimating a Money–Time Threshold." *Food Policy* **36**(2): 101–107.

Davis, G., and W. You (2013). "Estimates of Returns to Scale, Elasticity of Substitution, and the Thrifty Food Plan Meal Poverty Rate From a Direct Household Meal Production Function." *Food Policy* **43**: 204–212.

De Castro, J. (1994). "Family and Friends Produce Greater Social Facilitation of Food Intake Than Other Companions." *Physiol Behav* **56**: 445–455.

De Graaf, C., and F. Kok (2010). "Slow Food, Fast Food, and the Control of Food Intake." *Nature Rev Endo* **6**(5): 290–293.

Deaton, A. (2002). "Policy Implications of the Gradient of Health and Wealth." *Health Affairs* **21**(2): 13–30.

Deng, X., and R. Srinivasan (2013). "When Do Transparent Packages Increase (or Decrease) Food Consumption?" *J Mkting* **77**: 104–117.

Desrochers, P.m and H. Shimizu (2012). *The Locavore's Dilemma: In Praise of the 10,000-Mile Diet*. New York: Public Affairs.

DeVol, R., and A. Bedroussian. (2007). "An Unhealthy America: The Economic Burden of Chronic Disease." Retrieved September 3, 2014, from http://www.milkeninstitute.org/publications/publications.taf?function=detail&ID=38801018&cat=ResRep.

Dharmasena, S., and O. Capps Jr. (2012). "Intended and Unintended Consequences of a Proposed National Tax on Sugar-Sweetened Beverages to Combat the US Obesity Problem." *Health Econ* **21**(6): 669–694.

Dharmasena, S., G. Davis, and O. Capps Jr. (2014). "Partial Versus General Equilibrium Calorie and Revenue Effects Associated With a Sugar-Sweetened Beverage Tax." *J Agri and Res Econ* **39**(2): 157–173.

Dodd, M. (2014). "Intertemporal Discounting as a Risk Factor for High BMI: Evidence From Australia, 2008." *Econ Hum Biol* **12**: 83–97.

Dollahite, J., D. Kenkel, and C. Thompson (2008). "An Economic Evaluation of the Expanded Food and Nutrition Education Program." *J Nutr Educ Behav* **40**(3): 134–143.

Drewnowski, A., and N. Darmon (2005). "The Economics of Obesity: Dietary Energy Density and Energy Cost." *Am J Clin Nutr* **82**(1 Suppl): 265S–273S.

Drewnowski, A., and S. Specter (2004). "Poverty and Obesity: The Role of Energy Density and Energy Costs." *Am J Clin Nutr* **79**(1): 6–16.

Drichoutis, A., P. Lazaridis, and R. Nayga (2006). "Consumers' Use of Nutritional Labels: A Review of Research Studies and Issues." *Academy Mkting Sci Rev* **9**(9): 1–22.

Edelman, S. (2008). *Computing the Mind: How the Mind Really Works*. Oxford. UK. Oxford University Press.

Epstein, D., A. Sherwood, P. Smith, L. Craighead, C. Caccia, P. Lin, M. Babyak, J. Johnson, A. Hinderliter, and J. Blumenthal (2012). "Determinants and Consequences of Adherence to the DASH Diet in African American and White Adults With High Blood Pressure: Results From the Encore Trial." *J Acad Nutr Diet* **112**(11): 1763–1773.

Epstein, L., H. Jankowiak, R. Paluch, M. Koffarnus, and W. Bickel (2014). "No Food for Thought: Moderating Effects of Delay Discounting and Future Time Perspective on the Relation Between Income and Food Insecurity." *Am J Clin Nutr* **100**: 884–890.

Epstein, S. (1990). Cognitive-Experiential Self-Theory. *Handbook of Personality Theory and Research*. L.A. Pervin, ed. New York: Guilford, pp. 165–192.

Ervin, R. (2011). "Healthy Eating Index—2005 Total and Component Scores For Adults Aged 20 and Over: National Health and Nutrition Examination Survey, 2003-2004." *Natl Health Stat Report* (44): 1–9.

Evans, J. (1984). "Heuristic and Analytic Processes in Reasoning." *Br J Psych* **75**(4): 451–468.

Fedoroff, J., J. Polivy, and C. Herman (2003). "The Specificity of Restrained Versus Unrestrained Eaters' Responses to Food Cues: General Desire to Eat, or Craving For the Cued Food?" *Appetite* **41**: 7–13.

Fehr, E., and A. Rangel (2011). "Neuroeconomic Foundations of Economic Choice- Recent Advances." *J Econ Perspect* **25**(4): 3–30.

Ferdman, R. (2015). The Chipotle Effect: Why America Is Obsessed With Fast Casual. *The Washington Post.* Feb. 2, 2015. https://www.washingtonpost.com/news/wonk/wp/2015/02/02/the-chipotle-effect-why-america-is-obsessed-with-fast-casual-food/

Finkelstein, E., L. Kiersten, B. Strombotne, N. Chan, and J. Krieger (2011). "Mandatory Menu Labeling in One Fast-Food Chain in King County, Washington." *Am J Prev Med* **40**: 122–127.

Finkelstein, E., C. Zhen, M. Bilger, J. Nonnemaker, A. Farooqui, and J. Todd (2013). "Implications of A Sugar-Sweetened Beverage (SSB) Tax When Substitutions to Non-Beverage Items Are Considered." *J Health Econ* **32**(1): 219–239.

Fletcher, J. (2011). Is Healthy Food Really Profitable? *QSR Magazine.* Dec., 2011. https://www.qsrmagazine.com/health/healthy-food-really-profitable

Frazao, E. (1999). "America's Eating Habits: Changes and Consequences." *Agriculture Information Bulletin, U.S. Department of Agriculture* (750).

Frederick, S., G. Loewenstein, and T. O'Donoghue (2002). "Time Discounting and Time Preference: A Critical Review." *J Econ Lit* **40**(2): 351–401.

Freedhoff, Y. (2014). "The Food Industry Is Neither Friend, Nor Foe, Nor Partner." *Obesity Rev* **15**(1): 6–8.

Freedman, D. (2014, July/August). How Junk Food Can End Obesity. *The Atlantic* **23**. http://www.theatlantic.com/magazine/archive/2013/07/how-junk-food-can-end-obesity/309396/

Fundenberg, D. (2006). "Advancing Beyond "Advances in Behavioral Economics"." *J Econ Lit* **44**(3): 694–711.

Gigerenzer, G., and W. Gaissmaier (2011). "Heuristic Decision Making." *Ann Rev Psych* **62**: 451–482.

Glanz, K., M. Basil, E. Maibach, J. Goldberg, and D. Snyder (1998). "Why Americans Eat What They Do: Taste, Nutrition, Cost, Convenience, and Weight Control Concerns as Influences on Food Consumptions." *J Am Diet Assoc* **98**(10): 1118–1126.

Glanz, K., K. Resnicow, J. Seymour, K. Hoy, H. Stewart, M. Lyons, and J. Goldberg (2007). "How Major Restaurant Chains Plan Their Menus: The Role of Profit, Demand, and Health." *Am J Prev Med* **32**(5): 383–388.

Glanz, K., B. Rimer, and K. Viswanath (2008). *Health Behavior and Health Education.* San Francisco, CA: Jossey-Bass.

Glimcher, P., and A. Rustichini (2004). "Neuroeconomics: The Consilience of Brain and Decision." *Science* **306**(5695): 447–452.

Gold, M., J. Siegal, L. Russell, and M. Weinstein (1996). *Cost-Effectiveness in Health and Medicine.* New York: Oxford University Press.

Gootman, J., J. McGinnis, and V. Kraak (2006). *Food Marketing to Children and Youth :: Threat or Opportunity?* Washington, DC: National Academies Press.

Green, L., J. Myerson, D. Lichtman, S. Rosen, and A. Fry (1996). "Temporal Discounting in Choice Between Delayed Rewards: The Role of Age and Income." *Psych and Aging* **11**(1): 79–84.

Gregory, C., and P. Deb (2015). "Does SNAP Improve Your Health?" *Food Policy* **50**: 11–19.

Gregory, C., M. Ver Ploeg, M. Andrews, and A. Coleman-Jensen (2013). *Supplemental Nutrition Assistance Program (SNAP) Participation Leads to Modest Changes in Diet Quality.* U.S. Department of Agriculture.

Grimm, K., J. Foltz, H. Blanck, and K. Scanlon (2012). "Household Income Disparities in Fruit and Vegetable Consumption by State and Territory: Results of the 2009 Behavioral Risk Factor Surveillance System." *J Acad Nutr and Diet* **112**(12): 2014–2021.

Grossman, M. (1972). "On the Concept of Health Capital and the Demand For Health." *J Pol Econ* **80**(2): 223–255.

Gundersen, C., B. Kreider, and J. Pepper (2011). "The Economics of Food Insecurity in the United States." *App Econ Perspec and Policy* **33**(3): 281–303.

Guthrie, J., L. Mancino, and C. J. Lin (2015). "Nudging Consumers Toward Better Food Choices: Policy Approaches to Changing Food Consumption Behaviors." *Psych and Mkting* **32**(5): 501–511.

Haack, S., and C. Byker (2014). "Recent Population Adherence to and Knowledge of United States Federal Nutrition Guides, 1992–2013: A Systematic Review." *Nutr Rev* **72**(10): 613–626.

Hanks, A., D. Just, L. Smith, and B. Wansink (2012). "Healthy Convenience: Nudging Students Toward Healthier Choices in the Lunchroom." *J Pub Health* **34**(3): 370–376.

Harris, J., J. Bargh, and K. Brownell (2009). "Priming Effects of Television Food Advertising on Eating Behavior." *Health Psych* **28**(4): 404–413.

Harris, J., M. Schwartz, C. Munsell, C. Dembek, S. Liu, M. LoDolce, A. Heard, F. Fleming-Milici, and B. Kidd (2013). *Fast Food Facts 2013: Measuring Progress in Nutrition and Marketing to Children and Teens.* Yale Rudd Center for Food Policy & Obesity.

Harris, J., M. Weinberg, M. Schwartz, G. Ross, J. Ostroff, and K. Brownell (2010). *Trends in Television Food Advertising: Progress in Reducing Unhealthy Marketing to Young People?* Rudd Center.

Hastings, G., M. Stead, L. McDermott, A. Forsyth, A. MacKintosh, M. Rayner, C. Godfrey, M. Caraher, and K. Angus (2003). *Review of Research on the Effects of Food Promotion to Children.* Citeseer.

Hayden, G., and S. Ellis (2007). "Law and Economics After Behavioral Economics." *Univ KS Law Rev* **55**: 629–675.

Healthy People, 2020. (2015). "Disparities." Retrieved July 20, 2014, from http://www.healthypeople.gov/2020/about/foundation-health-measures/Disparities.

Hearst, M., L. Harnack, K. Bauer, A. Earnest, S. French, and J. Oakes (2013). "Nutritional Quality at Eight US Fast-Food Chains: 14-Year Trends." *Am J Prev Med* **44**(6): 589–594.

Herman, C., and J. Polivy (2005). "Normative Influences On Food Intake." *Phys and Behav* **86**(5): 762–772.

Hewstone, M., M. Rubin, and H. Willis (2002). "Intergroup Bias." *Ann Rev Clin Psych* **53**: 575–604.

Hieke, S., and C. Taylor (2012). "A Critical Review of the Literature on Nutritional Labeling." *J Cons Affairs* **46**(1): 120–156.

Hiza, H., K. Casavale, P. Guenther, and C. Davis (2013). "Diet Quality of Americans Differs by Age, Sex, Race/Ethnicity, Income, and Education Level." *J Acad Nutr and Diet* **113**(2): 297–306.

Holland, P. (1986). "Statistics and Causal Inference." *J Am Stat Assoc* **81**(396): 945–960.

Holmes, A., E. Serrano, J. Machin, T. Duestsch, and G. Davis (2013). "Effect of Different Children's Menu Labeling Designs on Family Purchases." *Appetite* **62**: 198–202.

Hoppe, R. (2014). *Structure and Finances of UD Farms: Family Farm Report, 2014 Edition,* USDA Economic Research Service, EIB.

Huffpost (July 8, 2013). "Agricultural Subsidies Promote Obesity, Charges New Study." http://www.huffingtonpost.com/2013/07/18/agriculture-subsidies-obesity_n_3607481.html

Husted, B., and J. de Jesus Salazar (2006). "Taking Friedman Seriously: Maximizing Profits and Social Performance*." *J Mgmt. Stud* **43**(1): 75–91.

Interagency Board for Nutrition Monitoring and Related Research (2000). *Nutrition Monitoring in the United States: The Directory of Federal and State Nutrition Monitoring and Related Research Activities.* K. Bialostosky, ed. Hyattsville, MD.

Jensen, M. (2002). "Value Maximization, Stakeholder Theory, and the Corporate Objective Function." *Bus Ethics Quarterly* **12**(2): 235–256.

Johnston, R., J. Poti, and B. Popkin (2014). "Eating and Aging: Trends in Dietary Intake Among Older Americans From 1977–2010." *J Nutr Health Aging* **18**(3): 234–242.

Jordan, L., J. Lee, and S. Yen (2004). "Do Dietary Intakes Affect Search for Nutrient Information on Food Labels?" *Soc Sci Med* **59**: 1955–1967.

Joy, A., V. Pradhan, and G. Goldman (2006). Cost-Benefit Analysis Conducted for Nutrition Education in California. *California Agriculture.* **60**: 185–191.

Just, D., and B. Wansink (2009). "Smarter Lunchrooms: Using Behavioral Economics to Improve Meal Selection." *Choices* **24**(3): 1–7.

Kahneman, D. (2011). *Thinking Fast and Slow.* New York. Farrar, Straus and Giroux.

Kentucky Fried Chicken (2014). "KFC Nutrition Guide." Retrieved Summer 2014 from http://www.kfc.com/nutrition/pdf/kfc_nutrition.pdf.

Keynes, J.N. (1917). *The Scope and Method of Political Economy.* 4th Ed. MacMillan. London.

Kim, D., and I. Kawachi (2006). "Food Taxation and Pricing Strategies to 'Thin Out' the Obesity Epidemic." *Am J Prev Med* **30**(5): 430–437.

Kinnucan, H., H. Xiao, C. Hsia, and J. Jackson (1997). "Effects of Health Information and Generic Advertising on US Meat Demand." *Am J Agr Econ* **79**(1): 13–23.

Kirkpatrick, S., K. Dodd, J. Reedy, and S. Krebs-Smith (2012). "Income and Race/Ethnicity Are Associated With Adherence to Food-Based Dietary Guidance Among US Adults and Children." *J Acad Nutr Diet* **112**(5): 624–635.

Kivi, P., and J. Shogren (2010). "Second Order Ambiguity in Very Low Probability Risks: Food Safety Valuation." *J Agr Res Econ* **35**(3): 443–456.

Kool, W., and M. Botvinick (2014). "A Labor/Leisure Tradeoff in Cognitive Control." *J Exp Psych* **143**(1): 131–141.

Kool, W., J. McGuire, Z. Rosen, and M. Botvinick (2010). "Decision Making and the Avoidance of Cognitive Demand." *J Exp Psych* **139**(4): 665–682.

Koplan, J., and K. Brownell (2010). "Response of the Food and Beverage Industry to the Obesity Threat." *JAMA* 304(13): 1487–1488.

Kraak, V., M. Story, E. Wartella, and J. Ginter (2011). "Industry Progress to Market a Healthful Diet to American Children and Adolescents." *Am J Prev Med* **41**(3): 322–333.

Kuhn, T. (1993). Reflections on My Critics. *Criticism and the Growth of Knowledge.* I. Lakatos and A. Musgrave, eds. Cambridge: Cambridge University Press.

Kurzban, R., A. Duckworth, J. Kable, and J. Myers (2013). "An Opportunity Cost Model of Subjective Effort and Task Performance." *Behav and Brain Sci* **36**(6): 661–679.

Lachat, C., E. Nago, R. Verstraeten, D. Roberfroid, J. Van Camp, and P. Kolsteren (2012). "Eating Out of Home and Its Association With Dietary Intake: A Systematic Review of the Evidence." *Obesity Reviews* **13**(4): 329–346.

Lehner, P., L. Adelman, B. Cheikes, and M. Brown (2008). "Confirmation Bias in Complex Analyses." *Systems, Man and Cybernetics, Part A: Systems and Humans, IEEE Transactions* **38**(3): 584–592.

Leung, C., E. Epel, L. Ritchie, P. Crawford, and B. Laraia (2014). "Food Insecurity Is Inversely Associated With Diet Quality of Lower-Income Adults." *J Acad Nutr Diet* **114**(12): 1943–1953.

Levin, I., and G. Gaeth (1988). "How Consumers Are Affected by the Framing of Attribute Information Before and After Consuming the Product." *J Cons Res* **15**: 374–378.

Levin, I.P., J. Schreiber, M. Lauriola, and G.J. Gaeth (2002). "A Tale of Two Pizzas: Building Up From a Basic Product Versus Scaling Down From a Fully-Loaded Product." *Market Lett* **13**(4): 335–344.

Levine, D. (2012). *Is Behavioral Economics Doomed? The Ordinary Versus the Extraordinary*.Cambridge UK Open Book Publishers.

Li, Y., B. Mills, G. Davis, and E. Mykerezi (2014). "Child Food Insecurity and the Food Stamp Program: What a Difference Monthly Data Make." *Soc Serv Rev* **88**(2): 322–348.

Lin, B., and J. Guthrie (2012). *Nutritional Quality of Food Prepared At Home and Away From Home, 1977–2008*. Washington, DC: U.S. Department of Agriculture, Economic Research Service.

Lin, B., T. Smith, J. Lee, and K. Hall (2011). "Measuring Weight and Outcomes for Obesity Intervention Strategies: The Case of a Sugar-Sweetened Beverage Tax." *Econ Hum Biol* **9**: 329–341.

Lipsky, L. (2009). "Are Energy-Dense Foods Really Cheaper? Reexamining the Relation Between Food Price and Energy Density." *Am J Clin Nutr* **90**: 1397–1401.

Lobstein, T., and S. Dibb (2005). "Evidence of a Possible Link Between Obesogenic Food Advertising and Child Overweight." *Obes Rev* **6**: 203–206.

Loewenstein, G. (1996). "Out of Control: Visceral Influences on Behavior." *Organ Behr and Hum Dec* **65**(3): 272–292.

Loewenstein, G., T. O'Donoghue, and M. Rabin (2003). "Projection Bias in Predicting Future Utility." *Quart J Econ* **118**(4): 1209–1248.

Loewenstein, G., and P. Ubel (2010). "Economics Behaving Badly." Op-Ed page. *New York Times*, July, 14.

Lusk, J. (2013). *The Food Police: A Well-Fed Manifesto About the Politics of Your Plate*. New York: Random House.

Lusk, J. (2014). "Are You Smart Enough to Know What to Eat? A Critique of Behavioural Economics as Justification for Regulation." *Eur Rev Agr Econ* **41**(3): 355–373.

Mabli, J., and J. Ohls (2015). "Supplemental Nutrition Assistance Program Participation Is Associated With an Increase in Household Food Security in a National Evaluation." *J Nutr* **145**(2): 344–351.

Mancino, L., and J. Kinsey (2008). *Is Dietary Knowledge Enough? Hunger, Stress, and Other Roadblocks to Healthy Eating*. Economic Research Report. Washington, DC.

Marshall, A. (1920). *Principles of Economics*, 8th ed. New York: The Macmillan Company.

Marteau, T., G. Hollands, and P. Fletcher (2012). "Changing Human Behavior to Prevent Disease: The Importance of Targeting Automatic Processes." *Science* **337**(6101): 1492–1495.

McCaffree, J. (2001). "Helping Clients Sort Out and Apply Media Messages." *J Am Diet Assoc* **1**(101):41.

McDonald's (2014). "Nutrition Choices." Retrieved Summer 2014 from http://www.mcdon-alds.com/us/en/food/food_quality/nutrition_choices.html.

McWilliams, A., and D. Siegel (2001). "Corporate Social Responsibility: A Theory of the Firm Perspective." *Acad Mgmt Review* **26**(1): 117–127.

Melby, M., and W. Takeda (2014). "Lifestyle Contraints, Not Inadequate Nutrition Education, Cause Gap Between Breakfast Ideals and Realities Among Japanese in Tokyo." *Appetite* **72**(1): 37–49.

Mill, J. (1950). *John Stuart Mill's Philosophy of Scientific Method*. The Hafner Library of Classics, E. Nagel, ed. New York: Hafner Publishing Company.

Mills, S., L. Tanner, and J. Adams (2013). "Systematic Literature Review of the Effects of Food and Drink Advertising on Food and Drink-Related Behaviour, Attitudes and Beliefs in Adult Populations." *Obesity Rev* **14**: 303–314.

Mischel, W., Y. Shoda, and M. Rodriguez (1989). "Delay of Gratification in Children." *Science* **244**(4907): 933–938.

Mitchell, G. (2005). "Libertarian Paternalism Is an Oxymoron." *Northwestern Univ Law Review* **99**(3):1248-1277.

Monsivais, P., A. Aggarwal, and A. Drewnowski (2014). "Time Spent on Home Food Preparation and Indicators of Healthy Eating." *Am J Prev Med* **47**(6): 796–802.

Moss, M. (2014). *Salt, Sugar, Fat: How the Food Giants Hooked Us*. New York: Random House Trade Paperbacks.

Mothersbaugh, D., R. Herrmann, and R. Warland (1993). "Perceived Time Pressure and Recommended Dietary Practices: The Moderating Effect of Knowledge of Nutrition." *J Cons Affairs* **27**(1): 106–126.

Muennig, P. (2007). *Cost-Effectiveness Analysis in Health: A Practical Approach*. San Francisco. John Wiley & Sons.

Mullainathan, S., and E. Shafir (2013). *Scarcity: Why Having Too Little Means So Much*. New York: Times Books.

Muraven, M., and R. Baumeister (2000). "Self-Regulation and Depletion of Limited Resources: Does Self-Control Resemble a Muscle?" *Psych Bulletin* **126**(2): 247–259.

National Osteoporosis Foundation (2014). "54 Million Americans Affected by Osteoporosis and Low Bone Mass." Retrieved July 20, 2014, from http://nof.org/news/2948.

Neuberger, E., and W. Duffy (1976). *Comparative Economic Systems: A Decision-Making Approach*. Boston: Allyn and Bacon Inc.

Neumann, N., and U. Bockenholt (2014). "A Meta-Analysis of Loss Aversion in Product Choice." *J Retailing* **90**(2): 182–197.

Neumann, P., J. Cohen, and M. Weinstein (2014). "Updating Cost-Effectiveness—The Curious Resilience of the $50,000-Per-QALY Threshold." *N Engl J Med* **371**(9): 796–797.

Newsday (April 22, 2015). "Mystery of Chipotle's Rising Tortilla Costs Solved." From http://www.newsday.com/business/mystery-of-chipotle-s-rising-tortilla-costs-is-solved-1.10314738.

Nguyen, A., R. Moser, and W. Chou (2014). "Race and Health Profiles in the United States: An Examination of the Social Gradient Through the 2009 Chis Adult Survey." *Public Health* **128**(12): 1076–1086.

Nickerson, R. (1998). "Confirmation Bias: A Ubiquitous Phenomenon in Many Guises." *Rev Gen Psychol* **2**(2): 175–220.

Nijs, I., P. Muris, A. Euser, and I. Franken (2010). "Differences in Attention to Food and Food Intake Between Overweight/Obese and Normal-Weight Females Under Conditions of Hunger and Satiety." *Appetite* **54**: 243–254.

NuVal. (2015). "NuVal 1-100. Nutrition Made Easy." Retrieved July 1, 2015, from https://www.nuval.com/.

Nwankwo, T., S. Yoon, V. Burt, and Q. Gu (2013). *Hypertension Among Adults in the US: National Health and Nutrition Examination Survey, 2011-2012. NCHS Data Brief, No. 133.* National Center for Health Statistics, Centers for Disease Control and Prevention, U.S. Dept. of Health and Human Services. Hyattsville, MD.

Obbagy, J., M. Condrasky, L. Roe, J. Sharp, and B. Rolls (2011). "Chefs' Opinions About Reducing the Calorie Content of Menu Items in Restaurants." *Obesity* **19**(2): 332–337.

O'Donoghue, E., R. Hoppe, D. Banker, and P. Korb (2009). *Exploring Alternative Farm Definitions: Implications For Agricultural Statistics and Program Eligibility.* Economic Research Service, Paper (49).

O'Donoghue, T., and M. Rabin (2006). "Optimal Sin Taxes." *J Public Econ* **90**: 1825–1849.

Ogden, C., M. Lamb, B. Kit, and K. Flegal (2014). "Prevalence of Childhood and Adult Obesity in the United States 2011–2012." *J Am Med Assoc* **311**(8): 806–814.

Okrent, A., and J. Alston (2012). "The Effects of Farm Commodity and Retail Food Policies on Obesity and Economic Welfare in the United States." *Am J Agr Econ* **94**(3): 611–646.

Okrent, A., and J. MacEwan (2014). "The Effects of Prices, Advertising, Expenditures, and Demographics on Demand for Nonalcoholic Beverages." *Agr and Res Econ Rev* **43**(1): 31–52.

Oliver, J. (2012). *Jamie's 15 Minute Meals.* UK: Michael Joseph.

Payne, J., J. Bettman, and E. Johnson (1993). *The Adaptive Decision Maker.* New York. Cambridge University Press.

Persky, J. (1993). "Retrospectives: Consumer Sovereignty." *J Econ Perspec* **7**(1): 183–191.

Pianin, E. (July 25, 2012). Billions in Tax Dollars Subsidize Junk Food Industry. *The Fiscal Times.* http://www.thefiscaltimes.com/Articles/2012/07/25/Billions-in-Tax-Dollars-Subsidize-Junk-Food-Industry

Pocheptsova, A., O. Amir, R. Dhar, and R. Baumeister (2009). "Deciding Without Resources: Resource Depletion and Choice in Context." *J Mkting* **46**: 344–355.

Poincaré, H. (1905). *Science and Hypothesis.* New York: The Walter Scott Publishing Co.

Poirier, D. (1995). *Intermediate Statistics and Econometrics: A Comparative Approach.* Cambridge, MA: The MIT Press.

Pollan, M. (2003). "The (Agri)Cultural Contradictions of Obesity." *New York Times,* Oct. 12.

Pollan, M. (2006). *The Omnivore's Dilemma: A History of Four Meals.* London: Penguin Books, Ltd.

Poti, J., M. Mendez, S. Ng, and B. Popkin (2015). "Is the Degree of Food Processing and Convenience Linked With the Nutritional Quality of Foods Purchased by US Households?" *Am J Clin Nutr* **101**(6): 1251–1262.

Powell, L., and Y. Bao (2009). "Food Prices, Access to Food Outlets and Child Weight." *Econ Hum Biol* **7**: 64–72.

Powell, L., J. Chriqui, R. Wada, and F. Chaloupka (2013). "Assessing the Potential Effectiveness of Food and Beverage Taxes and Subsidies For Improving Public Health: A Systematic Review of Prices, Demand and Body Weight Outcomes." *Obes Rev* **14**: 110–128.

Rabin, M. (2013a). "An Approach to Incorporating Psychology Into Economics." *Am Econ Rev* **103**(3): 617–622.

Rabin, M. (2013b). "Incorporating Limited Rationality Into Economics." *J Econ Lit* **51**(2): 528–543.

Raghunathan, R., R. Naylor, and W. Hoyer (2006). "The Unhealthy = Tasty Intuition and Its Effects on Taste Inferences, Enjoyment, and Choice of Food Products." *J Mkting* **70**(4): 170–184.

Rajgopal, R., R. Cox, M. Lamburm and E. Lewis (2002). "Cost-Benefit Analysis Indicates the Positive Economic Benefits of the Expanded Food and Nutrition Education Program Related to Chronic Disease Prevention." *J Nutr Educ Behav* **34**(1): 26–37.

Rangel, A. (2013). "Regulation of Dietary Choice by the Decision-Making Circuitry." *Nature Neuroscience* **16**(12): 1717–1724.

Rao, M., A. Afshin, G. Singh and D. Mozaffarian (2013). "Do Healthier Foods and Diet Patterns Cost More Than Less Healthy Options? A Systematic Review and Meta-Analysis." *BMJ Open* **3**(12): e004277.

Ray, R. (2006). *Classic Thirty-Minute Meals*. New York: Lake Isle Press.

Read, D., and B. Van Leeuwen (1998). "Predicting Hunger: The Effects of Appetite and Delay on Choice." *Organ Behav Hum Dec* **76**(2): 189–205.

Reedy, J., and S. Krebs-Smith (2010). "Dietary Sources of Energy, Solid Fats, and Added Sugars Among Children and Adolescents in the United States." *J Am Diet Assoc* **110**(10): 1477–1484.

Rickard, B., J. Liaukonyte, H. Kaiser, and T. Richards (2011). "Consumer Response to Commodity-Specific and Broad-Based Promotion Programs for Fruits and Vegetables." *Am J Agr Econ* **93**(5): 1312–1327.

Rickard, B., A. Okrent, and J. Alston (2013). "How Have Agricultural Policies Influenced Caloric Consumption in the United States?" *Health Econ* **22**(3): 316–339.

Rizzo, M., and D. Whitma (2009). "Knowledge Problem of New Paternalism." *Brigham Young Univ Law Review*: **209**(4):905–968.

Roberto, C., P. Larsen, H. Agnew, J. Baik, and K. Brownell (2010). "Evaluating the Impact of Menu Labeling On Food Choices and Intake." *Am J Public Health* **100**: 312–318.

Rollins, B., K. Dearing, and L. Epstein (2010). "Delay Discounting Moderates the Effect of Food Reinforcement on Energy Intake Among Non-Obese Women." *Appetite* **55**: 420–425.

Rolls, B., E. Morris and L. Roe (2002). "Portion Size of Food Affects Energy Intake in Normal-Weight and Overweight Men and Women." *Am J Clin Nutr* **76**(6): 1207–1213.

Rothman, A., P. Sherran and W. Wood (2009). "Reflective and Automatic Processes in the Initiation and Maintenance of Dietary Change." *Ann Behav Med* **38**(1): 4–17.

Rothman, R., R. Housam, H. Weiss, D. Davis, R. Gregory, T. Gebretsadik, A. Shintani and T. Elasy (2006). "Patient Understanding of Food Labels, The Role of Literacy and Numeracy." *Am J Prev Med* **31**(5): 391–398.

Ruhm, C. (2012). "Understanding Overeating and Obesity." *J Health Econ* **31**(6): 781–796.

Rusmevichientong, P., N. Streletskaya, W. Amatyakulm and H. Kaiser (2014). "The Impact of Food Advertisements on Changing Eating Behaviors: An Experimental Study." *Food Policy* **44**: 59–67.

Schachter, S., and L. Gross (1968). "Manipulated Time and Eating Behavior." *J Pers Soc Psychol* **10**: 98–106.

Scheibehenne, B., P. Todd, and B. Wansink (2010). "Dining in the Dark: The Importance of Visual Cues for Food Consumption and Satiety." *Appetite* **55**(3): 710–713.

Schuster, E., Z. Zimmerman, M. Engle, J. Smiley, E. Syversen, and J. Murray (2003). "Investing in Oregon's Expanded Food and Nutrition Education Program (EFNEP): Documenting Costs and Benefits." *J Nutr Educ Behav* **35**(4): 200–206.

Seeley, E. (1992). "Human Needs and Consumer Economics: The Implications of Maslow's Theory of Motivation For Consumer Expenditure Patterns." *J Socio-Econ* **21**(4): 303–324.

Sethuraman, R., G. Tellis, and R. Briesch (2011). "How Well Does Advertising Work? Generalizations From Meta-Analysis of Brand Advertising Elasticities." *J Mkting* **48**(3): 457–471.

Sheeran, P., P. Gollwitzer, and J. Bargh (2013). "Nonconscious Processes and Health." *Health Psych* **32**(5): 460–473.

Shiv, B., and A. Fedorikhin (1999). "Heart and Mind in Conflict: The Interplay of Affect and Cognition in Consumer Decision Making." *J Cons Res* **26**(3): 278–292.

Shulman, R., D. Rothman, K. Behar, and F. Hyder (2004). "Energetic Basis of Brain Activity: Implications for Neuroimaging." *Trends Neurosci* **27**(8): 489–495.

Smith, A. (1991). *An Inquiry Into the Nature and Causes of the Wealth of Nations.* New York: Alfred A. Knopf, Inc.

Smith, L., S. Ng, and B. Popkin (2013). "Trends in US Home Food Preparation and Consumption: Analysis of National Nutrition Surveys and Time Use Studies From 1965–1966 to 2007–2008." *Nutr J* **12**(1): 45.

Sobal, J., L. Khan, and C. Bisogni (1998). "A Conceptual Model of the Food and Nutrition System." *Social Sci Med* **47**(7): 853–863.

Sobal, J., and B. Wansink (2007). "Kitchenscapes, Tablescapes, Platescapes, and Food Scapes: Influences of Microscale Built Environments on Food Intake." *Environ Behav* **39**: 124–142.

Steinberg, L., S. Graham, L. O'Brien, J. Woolard, E. Cauffman, and M. Banich (2009). "Age Differences in Future Orientation and Delay Discounting." *Child Develop* **80**(1): 28–44.

Sterman, J. (1994). "Learning in and About Complex Systems." *Systems Dynamic Rev* **10**(2–3): 291–330.

Stewart, H., J. Hyman, E. Frazao, J. Buzby, and A. Carlson (2011). "Can Low-Income Americans Afford to Satisfy MyPyramid Fruit and Vegetable Guidelines?" *J Nutr Educ Behav* **43**(3):173–179.

Stigler, G., and G. Becker (1977). "De Gustibus Non Est Disputandum." *Am Econ Rev* **67**(2): 76–90.

Storey, M., and P. Anderson (2014). "Income and Race/Ethnicity Influence Dietary Fiber Intake and Vegetable Consumption." *Nutr Res* **34**(10): 844–850.

Story, M., M. Hamm, and D. Wallinga (2009). "Food Systems and Public Health: Linkages to Achieve Healthier Diets and Healthier Communities." *J Hunger and Envir Nutr* **4**(3–4): 219–224.

Strack, F., and R. Deutsch (2004). "Reflective and Impulsive Determinants of Social Behavior." *Person Social Psych Rev* **8**(3): 220–247.

Stroebele, N., and J. De Castro (2004). "Effect of Ambience on Food Intake and Food Choice." *Nutrition* **20**(9): 821–838.

Stuckler, D., and M. Nestle (2012). "Big Food, Food Systems, and Global Health." *PLoS Med* **9**(6): 678.

Sullivan, N., C. Hutcherson, A. Harris, and A. Rangel (2015). "Dietary Self-Control Is Related to the Speed With Which Attributes of Healthfulness and Tastiness Are Processed." *Psych Sci* **26**(2): 122–134.

Swartz, J., D. Braxton, and A. Viera (2011). "Calorie Menu Labeling on Quick-Service Restaurant Menus: An Updated Systematic Review of the Literature." *J Behav Nutr and Phys Act* **8**: 135.

Swinburn, B., V. Kraak, H. Rutter, S. Vandevijvere, T. Lobstein, G. Sacks, F. Gomes, T. Marshm and R. Magnusson (2015, June 20). "Strengthening of Accountability Systems to Create Healthy Food Environments and Reduce Global Obesity." *The Lancet* **385**(9986): 2534–2545.

Tandon, P., C. Zhou, N. Chan, P. Lozano, S. Couch, K. Glanz, J. Krieger, and B. Saelens (2011). "The Impact of Menu Labeling on Fast-Food Purchases for Children and Parents." *Am J Prev Med* **41**(4): 434–438.

Thaler, R. and C. Sunstein (2009). *Nudge: Improving Decisions About Health, Wealth, and Happiness*. New Haven, CT: Yale University Press.

Thorndike, A., L. Sonnenberg, J. Riis, S. Barraclough, and D. Levy (2012). "A 2-Phase Labeling and Choice Architecture Intervention to Improve Healthy Food and Beverage Choices." *Am J Public Health* **102**(3): 527–533.

Trefis Team (2014, June 23). How the Fast Casual Segment Is Gaining Market Share in the Restaurant Industry. *Forbes*. Available at http://www.forbes.com/sites/greatspeculations/2014/06/23/how-the-fast-casual-segment-is-gaining-market-share-in-the-restaurant-industry/

Tversky, A., and D. Kahneman (1991). "Loss Aversion in Riskless Choice: A Reference-Dependent Model." *Quart J Econ* **106**(4): 1039–1061.

U.S. Census Bureau (2007). "Survey of Current Business Owners." Retrieved Spring 2015 from http://www.census.gov/econ/sbo/.

U.S. Census Bureau (2012). "North American Industry Classification System." Retrieved Spring 2015 from http://www.census.gov/cgi-bin/sssd/naics/naicsrch?code=11411&search=2012%20NAICS%20Search.

U.S. Census Bureau, Business and Industry (2015). "Annual Wholesale and Retail Trade Data." Retrieved Spring 2015 from http://www.census.gov/econ/index.html.

U.S. Department of Agriculture, Agricultural Research Service. (2014). "National Nutrient Database For Standard Reference Release 27." Retrieved July 20, 2014, from http://ndb.nal.usda.gov/ndb/search/list.

U.S. Department of Agriculture, Center for Nutrition Policy and Promotion (2013). Diet Quality of Children Age 2–17 Years as Measured by the Healthy Eating Index, 2010. *Nutrition Insight 52*.

U.S. Department of Agriculture, Center for Nutrition Policy and Promotion (2014). "Choosemyplate.Gov." Retrieved July 20, 2014, from www.choosemyplate.gov.

U.S. Department of Agriculture, Center for Nutrition Policy and Promotion (2015). "Healthy Eating Index." Retrieved Spring 2015. http://www.cnpp.usda.gov/healthyeatingindex.

U.S. Department of Agriculture, Economic Research Service (2014c). "Food Expenditures, Table 1." Retrieved Summer 2014 from http://www.ers.usda.gov/data-products/food-expenditures.aspx.

U.S. Department of Agriculture, Economic Research Service (2014f). "Food Wholesaling." Retrieved Spring 2015 from http://www.ers.usda.gov/topics/food-markets-prices/retailing-wholesaling/wholesaling.aspx.

U.S. Department of Agriculture, Economic Research Service (2015). "Food Dollar Series." Retrieved Spring 2015 from http://www.ers.usda.gov/data-products/food-dollar-series.aspx.

U.S. Department of Agriculture, Economic Research Service (2015a). "Food Security in the US." Retrieved Spring 2015 from http://www.ers.usda.gov/topics/food-nutrition-assistance/food-security-in-the-us/survey-tools.aspx.

U.S. Department of Agriculture, Economic Research Service, Feed Grains Yearbook (2015). "Average Corn Prices Received by Farmers (Table 9)." Retrieved Spring 2015 from http://www.ers.usda.gov/datafiles/Feed_Grains_Yearbook_Tables/Domestic_and_International_Prices/FGYearbookTable09Full.htm.

U.S. Department of Agriculture, Economic Research Service, Food Dollar Series (2015). "Industry Group Series." Retrieved Spring 2015 from http://www.ers.usda.gov/data-products/food-dollar-series/food-dollar-application.aspx.

U.S. Department of Agriculture, Food and Nutrition Service. (2014). "Chicken and Cranberry Salad." *What's Cooking?* Retrieved Summer 2014 from www.usda.gov/whatscooking.

U.S. Department of Agriculture, Food and Nutrition Service SNAP-Ed (2015). "Supplemental Nutrition Assistance Program Education (Snap-Ed)." Retrieved July 1, 2015, from http://www.fns.usda.gov/snap/supplemental-nutrition-assistance-program-education-snap-ed.

U.S. Department of Agriculture, Food and Nutrition Service WIC (2015b). "WIC." Retrieved July 1, 2015, from http://www.fns.usda.gov/wic/women-infants-and-children-wic.

U.S. Department of Agriculture, National Agricultural Library. (2015). "DRI Tables and Application Reports." Retrieved July 1, 2015, from http://fnic.nal.usda.gov/dietary-guidance/dietary-reference-intakes/dri-tables-and-application-reports.

U.S. Department of Agriculture, National Agricultural Statistics Service (2011). "Agricultural Statistics." Washington, DC: U.S. Government Printing Office.

U.S. Department of Agriculture, National Institute of Food and Agriculture EFNEP (2015). "Expanded Food and Nutrition Education Program." Retrieved July 1, 2015, from http://nifa.usda.gov/program/expanded-food-and-nutrition-education-program-efnep.

U.S. Department of Agriculture, Nutrition Evidence Library (2014). "Nutrition Evidence Library." Retrieved Summer 2014 from http://www.nel.gov/.

U.S. Department of Health and Human Services (2010). *Dietary Guidelines For Americans 2010*, 7th ed. Washington, DC: U.S. Government Printing Office.

U.S. Department of Health and Human Services (2015). *Scientific Report of the 2015 Dietary Guidelines Advisory* Committee.

U.S. Food and Drug Administration (2015a). "Nutrition Facts Label Programs & Materials." Retrieved July 1, 2015, from http://www.fda.gov/Food/IngredientsPackagingLabeling/LabelingNutrition/ucm20026097.htm.

U.S. Food and Drug Administration (2015b). "Proposed Changes to the Nutrition Facts Label." Retrieved July 1, 2015, from http://www.fda.gov/Food/GuidanceRegulation/GuidanceDocumentsRegulatoryInformation/LabelingNutrition/ucm385663.htm.

Varian, H. (2006). *Intermediate Microeconomics*. New York: W.W. Norton & Company, Inc.

Vernarelli, J., D. Mitchell, B. Rolls, and T. Hartman (2013). "Methods for Calculating Dietary Energy Density in a Nationally Representative Sample." *Procedia Food Sci* 2: 68–74.

Vohs, K., and T. Heatherton (2000). "Self-Regulatory Failure: A Resource-Depletion Approach." *Psychol Sci* 11(3): 249–254.

Volkow, N., G. Wang, J. Fowler, J. Logan, M. Jayne, D. Franceschi, C. Wong, S. Gatley, A. Gifford, Y. Ding, and N. Pappas (2002). "'Nonhedonic' Food Motivation in Humans Involves Dopamine in the Dorsal Striatum and Methylphenidate Amplifies This Effect." *Synapse* **44**: 175–180.

Wadhera, D., and E. Capaldi-Phillips (2014). "A Review of Visual Cues Associated With Food on Food Acceptance and Consumption." *Eating Behaviors* **15**: 132–143.

Wang, D., C. Leung, Y. Li, E. Ding, S. Chiuve, F. Hu, and W. Willett (2014). "Trends in Dietary Quality Among Adults in the United States, 1999 Through 2010." *JAMA Intern Med* **174**(10): 1587–1595.

Wang, J., N. Novemsky, R. Dhar, and R. Baumeister (2010). "Trade-offs and Depletion in Choice." *J Mkting* **47**: 910–919.

Wansink, B. (2004). "Environmental Factors That Increase the Food Intake and Consumption Volume of Unknowing Consumers." *Ann Rev Nutr* **24**: 455–479.

Wansink, B. (2006). *Mindless Eating: Why We Eat More Than We Think.* New York: Bantam Books.

Wansink, B. (2014). *Slim by Design: Mindless Eating Solutions for Everyday Life.* New York: William Morrow.

Wansink, B., and J. Kim (2005). "Bad Popcorn in Big Buckets: Portion Size Can Influence Intake as Much as Taste." *J Nutr Educ Behav* **37**(5): 242–245.

Wansink, B., J. Painter, and Y. Lee (2006). "The Office Candy Dish: Proximity's Influence on Estimated and Actual Consumption." *Int J Obesity* **30**: 871–875.

Wansink, B. and J. Sobal (2007). "Mindless Eating: The 200 Daily Food Decisions We Overlook." *Environ Behav* **39**: 106.

Wansink, B., K. Van Ittersum and J. Painter (2005). "How Descriptive Food Names Bias Sensory Perceptions in Restaurants." *Food Qual Prefer* **16**(5): 393–400.

Wansink, B., K. van Ittersum and J. Painter (2006). "Ice Cream Illusions: Bowls, Spoons, and Self-Served Portion Sizes." *Am J Prev Med* **31**: 240–243.

Ward, B., J. Schiller, and R. Goodman (2014). "Multiple Chronic Conditions Among US Adults: A 2012 Update." *Preventing Chronic Disease* **11**: 130389.

Welch, N., S. McNaughton, W. Hunter, C. Hume, and D. Crawford (2009). "Is the Perception of Time Pressure a Barrier to Healthy Eating and Physical Activity Among Women?" *Public Health Nutr* **12**(7): 888–895.

Weller, R., E. Cook, K. Avsar, and J. Cox (2008). "Obese Women Show Greater Delay Discounting Than Healthy-Weight Women." *Appetite* **51**: 563–569.

Wells, H., and J. Buzby (2008). *Dietary Assessment of Major Trends in U.S. Food Consumption, 1970–2005.* Washington, DC: U.S. Department of Agriculture, Economic Research Service.

White, J. (2008). "Straight Talk About High-Fructose Corn Syrup: What It Is and What It Ain't." *Am J Clin Nutr* **88**(6): 1716S–1721S.

Wisdom, J., J. Downs, and G. Loewenstein (2010). "Promoting Healthy Choices: Information Versus Convenience." *Am Econ J: Appl Econ* **2**(2): 164–178.

Woods, A., E. Poloakoff, L. Kuenzel, R. Hodson, H. Gonda, J. Batchelor, G. Dijksterhuis, and A. Thomas (2011). "Effect of Background Noise on Food Perception." *Food Qual Prefer* **22**(1): 42–47.

World Cancer Research Fund, American Institute for Cancer Research (2007). *Food, Nutrition, Physical Activity, and the Prevention of Cancer: A Global Perspective.* Washington, DC: AICR.

Wu, H. (2015). "Unsavory Choices: The High Sodium Density of US Chain Restaurant Foods." *J Food Comp and Analysis* **40**: 103–105.

Wu, S., and A. Green. (2000). "Projection of Chronic Illness Prevalence and Cost Inflation." Retrieved August 26, 2014, from http://www.cdc.gov/chronicdisease/overview/index.htm.

Wu, H., and R. Sturm (2013). "What's on the Menu? A Review of the Energy and Nutritional Content of US Chain Restaurant Menus." *Public Health Nutr* **16**(01): 87–96.

Yach, D. (2014). "Food Industry: Friend or Foe?" *Obesity Rev* **15**(1): 2–5.

Yang, Y., G. Davis, and M. Muth (2015). "Beyond the Sticker Price: Including and Excluding Time in Comparing Food Prices." *Am J Clin Nutr* **102**(1): 165–171.

Zhen, C., E. Finkelstein, J. Nonnemaker, and S. Karns (2014). "Predicting the Effects of Sugar-Sweetened Beverage Taxes on Food and Beverage Demand in a Large Demand System." *Am J Agr Econ* **96**(1): 1–25.

Zimmerman, F., and S. Shimoga (2014). "The Effects of Food Advertising and Cognitive Load on Food Choices." *BMC Public Health* **14**: 342.

Zlatevska, N., C. Dubelaar, and S. Holden (2014). "Sizing Up the Effect of Portion Size on Consumption: A Meta-Analytic Review." *J Mkting* **78**(3): 140–154.

Zoellner, J., W. You, C. Connel, R. Smith-Ray, K. Allen, K. Tucker, B. Davy, and P. Estabrooks (2012). "Health Literacy Is Associated With Healthy Eating Index Scores and Sugar-Sweetened Beverage Intake: Findings from the Rural Lower Mississippi Delta." *J Am Diet Assoc* **111**: 1012–1020.

INDEX

Calories (*Cont.*)
  in proteins, 15
  recommendations, 13(table)
  tax impact on intake of, 204, 204(figure), 207
Camerer, C., 136
Cancer, 4–5, 6
  defined, 40
  dietary recommendations and, 38(table)
  number of deaths from, 4(table)
  overview of, 40
  overweight and obesity and, 37
Capital costs, 225, 226(table)
Capps, O., 208
Carbohydrates, 15
  consumption of relative to recommendations,
    31(table)
  defined, 5
  recommendations, 8(table)
Carlson, A., 84
Cartwright, Nancy, 104n2
Cash grain crops, 164
Cattle prices, 210, 211(figure)
Causal variables, 236, 237–38
Centers for Disease Control and Prevention, 37
Certainty weight, 116–17, 119, 120
Ceteris paribus
  ambiguity effect and, 128
  cognitive effort and, 143
  convenience and, 88
  defined, 77, 236
  downstream price-making firms and, 182
  importance in economic methodology,
    239, 242
  information and, 107
  intertemporal choice problem and, 115, 118
  market equilibrium and, 201
  obesity-corn subsidy correlation and, 217
  prices and, 77, 78, 82–83, 85, 196
  supply curve and, 174
  supply function and, 175
Chabris, C., 120, 137
Children
  advertising exposure and, 103, 109
  Healthy Eating Index on, 36
  overweight and obesity in, 37
  weight classifications for, 39(table)
Chloride, 6
Choice environment attributes, 124–25
Chou, S., 109
Chronic diseases
  dietary behavior and, 21(table)
  key nutrients in prevention of, 8–13(table)
  leading causes of death associated with, 4–5,
    4(table)
  nutrition role, 37–42
  prevalence of, 4

Chronic lower respiratory diseases, 4(table)
Cobalamin. *See* Vitamin B-12
Cobalt, 6
Cognitive effort
  minimized, 137
  as a moderating variable, 141–44, 143(figure)
Cognitive load, 137–38, 140
Cognitive resource allocation model,
    137–38, 143
Cognitive resource depletion, 137–38
"Cognitive tax," 141
Cold-hot empathy gap, 131–32
Competitive markets, 181–82, 193–218. *See
    also* Horizontally related markets; Market
    equilibrium; Vertically related markets
  imperfectly, 199, 199n2, 200
  perfectly, 199–201
Complements, 81, 83, 212
Compromise graph, 59, 69, 188
Computational theory of the brain, 136–37
Concomitants, 239
Confirmation effect, 129, 140, 158
Consumer sovereignty, 196, 201n3
Contour maps, 64–65
Convenience, 45, 88–90, 98. *See also* Time
    constraints
Copper, 6
Corn prices, 210, 211(figure)
Corn subsidies, 217
Coronary artery disease, 39
Corporate social responsibility (CSR), 147, 180,
    187–89, 188(figure), 190–91
  defined, 187
  strategic, 189, 190
Cost-benefit analysis (CBA), 222, 223, 224,
    229–32, 233–34
  defined, 229
  explained, 229–30
  pros and cons of, 231–32
  sample questions to answer for, 231(box)
Cost-effectiveness analysis (CEA), 222, 223,
    224, 232–34
  CBA as an extension of, 229, 231
  defined, 227
  explained, 227–28
  main limitation of, 229, 232–33
  pros and cons of, 232–33
Cost-effectiveness ratio (CER), 227–28, 233
Cost-identification analysis, 222, 223
  categories and types, 224–27, 226(table)
  defined, 224
Costs
  capital, 225, 226(table)
  direct, 225, 226(table)
  fixed (*see* Fixed costs)
  full (*see* Full cost)